A MINNESOTA DOCTOR'S
HOME REMEDIES
FOR
COMMON AND UNCOMMON
AILMENTS

A Minnesota Doctor's Home Remedies for Common and Uncommon Ailments

SECOND EDITION

JOHN E. EICHENLAUB, M. D.

PRENTICE-HALL, INC.   Englewood Cliffs, N.J.

Prentice-Hall International, Inc., *London*
Prentice-Hall of Australia, Pty. Ltd., *Sydney*
Prentice-Hall of Canada, Ltd., *Toronto*
Prentice-Hall of India Private Ltd., *New Delhi*
Prentice-Hall of Japan, Inc., *Tokyo*

© 1960, 1972 by
John E. Eichenlaub, M.D.

Library of Congress
Catalog Card Number: 75-179448

Printed in the United States of America
ISBN-0-13-584557-2
B&P

What This Book of Home Remedies Can Do for You

Very few people can go to a doctor for every misery, hurt or disorder. They have to weigh their difficulties against the time and money a physician's care may consume. Unless they have considerable distress, they often shrug off their complaints as burdens to be borne, and carry on as well as they can.

If that is what you sometimes have to do, the home remedies and other measures you find in this book will help you greatly. You can cure or relieve many ailments right in your own home, often without spending a dime for medicines or doctor care, or a minute waiting in a doctor's office. You can perk yourself up and boost your resistance to disease with simple, inexpensive home tonics. You can take definite countermeasures and maintain informed alertness against serious disease and deterioration. This book gives you exact directions for hundreds of simple home remedies, tonics, and counteractants with which to meet or avoid about 200 mild and serious ailments. It solves the recurring dilemma of physician's care *vs* stoical neglect by giving a third and often perfectly proper choice: well-managed, effective, convenient home measures.

Minnesota as home care center. An almost unique situation makes the Gopher State teem with tried and true home remedies. Although the isolation of old-time logging camps and wood-ringed farms has largely given way to modern progress, the hardy self-reliance of former days lives on. The people of this area usually go to the medicine chest instead of the nearest doctor when they get a sniffle or an ache. They can draw from all the traditions of Northern Europe as well as the scientific guidance of the medical centers at Rochester and Minneapolis. They have thousands of good doctors who are willing to correct and supplement home care instead of fighting it. No wonder Minnesotans get topnotch home care!

Another Scandinavian tradition is health promotion. No people in the world spend more effort building strength and vigor. When you think of Sweden, you think of calisthenics and gymnastic teams. Also, the thought of Finland brings the picture of steam-reddened bodies plunging into icy lakes for the sake of extra verve and vigor—a procedure that takes a world of courage, and could never have been discovered without true dedication to the pursuit of health. Constant awareness of health problems is part of this tradition: our University's cancer detection clinic has a long waiting list; our heart hospital has a large department devoted to preventive care; our School of Public Health includes a world-famous center for studying the bodily processes and the strains of ordinary life. Home remedies in Minnesota go beyond care for common ailments to energy-building, zest-restoring tonics unknown in many other areas and to procedures aimed at finding or preventing deadly ills.

YOU and your family need home remedies. I am sure that all of you suffer some of the illnesses and disorders considered in this book. Muscle and joint pains, indigestion, constipation, sex organ irritations, sluggish circulation etc.—few families escape all of these common disorders for even a month at a time. How many hours of misery could sound home treatment have saved you in the past year? How much lost time and patent medicine money? Perhaps you have even had expensive and uncomfortable doctor's care which proper home measures could have made unnecessary! You can take eight different steps to cure yourself of muscular backache and to keep it from troubling you again. You can rid yourself of corns and callouses forever with three simple measures. You can choose from 16 completely different approaches to joint misery, ranging from hormone-stimulating aspirin doses and warm flannel application to special massage, paraffin baths, and sleep-aiding braces. You can solve your constipation problem for good with the step-by-step home method outlined in Chapter Four. If rectal troubles have plagued you, learn how to distinguish hemorrhoids from splits or fissures and what curative measures you can take against each of these common miseries. Don't let aftermaths of motherhood like cystocoel and rectocoel build their discomforts through the years either: a slight change in the position you assume for emptying your bowel might save you the misery and expense of a later operation. And if you have had sex complaints—whether male or female—Chapter Six provides a broad assortment of remedies you can apply in the privacy of your own home. Other chapters deal with sinus trouble, stuffy nose, nasal crusts. These and other nose and throat discomforts yield to measures you can readily adopt. Home remedies give quick relief for many skin troubles, too, including conditions like eczema and psoriasis, for which no amount of prescription care brings permanent and lasting cure.

Even if you presently have none of these miseries or the dozens of others treated in the pages of this book, the chances are that you will have several occasions to use its helpful guidance during the next year. How many people live 12 months without a cold, without a scrape, bruise or burn, without a boil or skin eruption? You can apply the specific, concrete directions that this book offers to all of these and to many other common ailments. If you get a headache, for instance, you will find separate sections with exact treatment suggestions, for each of the seven commonest varieties of head pain. From itching scalp to ingrown toenail, you'll find exact, complete directions for handling home care of over 200 different disorders.

The world's most practical treatments! Most of the home remedies in this book call for substances and ingredients you can find in any household—hot and cold water, salt, baking soda, paraffin, and vinegar, for instance. Many of the others depend on standard medicine chest items like nose drops, rubbing alcohol, paregoric, castor oil, and petroleum jelly. You can buy almost all of the other materials needed without a prescription in your drugstore or dry goods store. In a few instances, when the materials available without prescription are in a less convenient form (e.g., non-prescription stomach-soothing suppositories vs. prescription pills) or are less economical (e.g., swallowed doses of relatively expensive ephedrine nose drops), the prescription equivalent has been included, too. You may want to ask your doctor to prescribe these remedies for your medicine chest when you next visit his office.

Tone up for vigorous living! Maybe it's the lure of 11,000 lovely lakes and 19 million acres of timberland, or maybe it's plain distaste for feeling old, but Minnesotans have more ways of toning up themselves than any other group I know. Several of their favorite techniques, detailed in Chapter Twelve, measurably increase your energy and vigor. Dr. Keys of Minnesota's Laboratory of Physiological Hygiene has been a front runner in investigations of health-improving foods, too. The concrete, three-step dietary program (described in Chapter Fourteen) for staving off hardened arteries and the other ravages once thought to be an inevitable part of old age is largely an outgrowth of his and other studies done right in this state. One thing I'll guarantee: you will definitely feel new zest and vigor through the fatigue-dispelling exercises, the stimulating home tonic methods and the nerve-soothing tranquilizing techniques that this book spells out. Procedures like the cold friction bath, the sheet bath, and the specially conducted rest period can lighten the burden of your daily life from this moment forth.

Counteract serious ailments and disorders. You have one advantage that even your doctor does not enjoy in fighting off illness: you can take action day by day to boost your resistance, and to ward off or detect the bare beginnings of disease. Action *right now* can cut your chance of suffering such conditions as the common cold, ulcers, skin infection, hardened arteries, coronary heart attacks, and even cancer. Learn to avoid these and many other health hazards with simple home measures! An ounce of prevention is worth more than a pound of cure. You can head off many plagues that no doctor on earth can stop once they have a grip on you. Corrective measures you can take right in your own home will add extra, youthful, vigorous, misery-free years to your lifespan. You'll find exact techniques outlined in full detail throughout this book.

Use doctor's care more effectively than ever before, too. You can make your doctor's care much more effective with home techniques, even when home remedies will not suffice. Learn to spot the illnesses and complications for which very prompt medical care is cheaper and better. Learn actual home techniques for identifying possibly serious health problems early, when your doctor's care will do you the most good. Learn how to make procedures like gall bladder surgery and the care of heart attacks much easier on you and much more effective. The measures advised in this book are realistic: they do not send you to your doctor for every sniffle. But they do reveal many ways in which you can get more help from your doctor without extra medical expense.

Home remedies, tonics and counteractants can help YOU. Make no mistake: a great many of the miseries and discomforts you have suffered will yield to home remedies. *You* can fight off illness and disease without undue expense or inconvenience. *You* can make yourself feel younger, more vigorous, and more cheerful by using home tonics. *You* can counteract threats of serious disease and deterioration with day-by-day home measures. Countless Minnesotans have tried the how-to techniques outlined in this book over a period of many years. Some of the country's finest doctors have helped weed out the old wives' tales from the genuine, useful remedies and have added their own wisdom to the fine distillate of Northern Europe's finest healing traditions. The results are all here, in this book. Won't you put its hundreds of practical remedies and tonics to work for you today?

John E. Eichenlaub, M.D.

Why This Second Edition?

Whenever a responsible author puts out a book, it's as good as he can make it. So why run it through the typewriter again for a Second Edition?

In the case of this book of my HOME REMEDIES, there are several reasons.

First, I have a better picture of your health needs. In the twelve years that have passed between editions of this book, a great many of its readers have written me, and hundreds of others have discussed the book with me during personal or live-audience contact I had with them. These readers have told me their circumstances, health problems and their resources. The spectrum of reader interest is broad, ranging from a missionary family in Africa who said that HOME REMEDIES was the only help they had with family illnesses for a year, to an elderly lady in a nursing home with doctors in constant attendance. They've told me what they hoped a new edition might cover. Children's doses, for instance—many readers have children or grandchildren and want to know whether the same techniques which work so well for adults will help youngsters too. Some of the difficulties they have asked me to cover are not here, either because the problem was unique or because I simply didn't have anything very helpful in the home remedy line to offer. But this edition has a very exact target at which to shoot, defined by the million or so readers of its predecessor edition. A substantial part of the new Second Edition meets special needs of which I became aware in this way.

Second, I know the subject better. An "authority" becomes a sort of clearing house for other people's information, from fascinating folklore to unpublished doctor-developed tips. Many of the methods I've added in this new edition—the fabulous ice therapy for sunburn, burns and scalds, for instance—came to me in this way.

Third, there's always progress and change. The old-time remedies remain the same—soaks and baths, massage and exercise, even paregoric and cough remedies—but new preparations, new viewpoints, and new circumstances make for new questions and new answers. When HOME REMEDIES was first published, no drug firm was making a cold pill which would shrink nose lining, so the book emphasized swallowed doses of ephedrine nose drops. Now, better materials are available without a prescription in cheaper, more convenient pill or capsule form. The first edition had nothing to say about "the pill" for contraception and how to handle its side effects such as irregularity and nausea, because "the pill" hadn't been invented. My advice on avoiding arterio-sclerosis by diet has held up remarkably well—it was duplicated almost word for word in the recommendations made by the Heart and Medical Associations many years after HOME REMEDIES was first published—but research has increased our understanding of this subject further year by year, and this book contains updated advice on it.

Last, there's the plain advantage of a second time around. I'm sure you've said to yourself at times: "If only I could scrap the whole thing and start over, I'd do a better job." I haven't changed every sentence in the Second Edition of this book, but the new or altered parts amount to pretty much of a clean sweep. There are two totally new chapters on family planning and home remedies during pregnancy, and literally dozens of new treatments and changes affecting every single chapter of this Second Edition of HOME REMEDIES.

At one stage of my medical career, I was associated with a doctor who always stopped at the end of each day's work to run his finger down the accounting list of his patients. A lot of people thought he was counting up the dollars, and criticized his "greed." But he had an entirely different point in mind. "Every day," he told me, "I count up the people who have come to see me, and I think what a great compliment it is, that all these people came to me with their problems—*me,* a poor boy from a ghetto whom most of them wouldn't have even looked at ten or fifteen years ago." I can't claim the ghetto background, but I share that same astonished feeling of pleasure in recognition and use. So let me close this brief introduction to this Second Edition with a salute to the millions of people who have read my books. Your acceptance of my offerings and use of my ideas has given me gratifications beyond what I can describe, and I most humbly thank you.

John E. Eichenlaub, M.D.

Contents

Muscular Backache. Hot showers with Figure 8 movement. Aspirin. Extra sleep support. Paraffin baths. Massage. How to conquer a tendency toward backache. Muscular Miseries, Cramps, and Charley Horses. How to relieve aching muscles. Neck and shoulder-arm pain. Muscle cramps. Foot troubles. How to trim corns and callouses. Relieving pressure to rid yourself of corns and callouses. Felt pads. Relief from blisters. Relief for painful arches. Adolescent arch strain. Tricks for taping. Tape for arch strain. Long-range help with arch troubles. Bunions. Ingrown toenail.

Joint Pains. Red, swollen joints. The hormone-stimulating aspirin dose. Red joints in children. Warm flannel. Diet. Bodily rest. Rest for sore joints. Motion-preserving exercises. Supported or flotation exercises. Cripple-cutting braces. Subsiding or smoldering joint trouble. Sore, stiff fingers. Aching arms, hips, or knees. Perpetual stiff neck. Stiff elbows, wrists, ankles, and toes. Diffuse joint trouble. Home whirlpool equipment. Hip, knee, and joint strain. Growing pains. **Neuritis, Bursitis, and Inflamed Leader**

Guides. Neuritis and neuralgia. Vitamin B₁. Massage with homemade wintergreen liniments. Flannel or cotton-knit protection. Bursitis. Pressure bandaging. Lightbulb heat. Hormone-boosting doses of aspirin. Rest. Leader guide inflammation. Splinting.

Diarrhea. The long fast. Bowel-flushing enemas. Fluid-restoring enemas. Diarrhea in children. Kaolin compounds. Paregoric. Stepwise reintroduction of foods. Salt. Allergic diarrhea. Antihistamines. Food and diarrhea records. Digestive Distress. Could this attack be appendicitis? Have attacks been sufficiently regular to suggest a serious underlying cause? Heartburn. Sick stomach. Sleeping tablets. Prescription nausea fighters. Gas and pressure pains. Suppositories. Spasm soothers. Low residue diet. Less milk. How to fight a tendency toward indigestion. Better teeth for good digestion. Food to fit your teeth. Take time to chew. Low acidity indigestion. Caffeine-spurred indigestion. Worms. Ulcers and Gastritis. Simplified ulcer-healing diet. Acid-absorbing milk. Antacids. Milk of magnesia. Convalescent diet. How to keep ulcer from coming back. Precautions under stress. Ulcer-dodging way of life. How much to depend on others emotionally and how much to let them depend on you. Learn to say, "No". Evade or rid yourself of resentment. Bilious Indigestion, and Gall Bladder Disease and Stone. Enemas and suppositories. Low fat diet. Bile salts. Laxative salts. Serious gall bladder trouble. How to make a gall bladder operation easier to bear.

Tight Bowels. Low-bulk diet. Gradually increase moist-bulk foods. Free yourself gradually of all bowel-regulating medicines. Constipation in Children. Constipation. How to empty your lower bowel efficiently. Exercise. Abdominal massage. Dodge dry bulk. Lessen tension. Temporary Relief Without Long-range Harm. Enemas. Disposable enema kits. Phosphates. Rid yourself of constipation worries. **Special Forms of Constipation.** Rectal accumulations. Blocked bowel.

Hemorrhoids. How to soothe clotted hemorrhoids. Irritated hemorrhoids. Increasing or newly formed hemorrhoids. Protruding hemorrhoids. When your doctor's help is worthwhile for hemorrhoids. **Rectal itching.** How to cure rectal dermatitis. Malt soup extract. When your doctor can help with rectal itching. **Pinworms.** Home check for pinworms. Doctor tests for pinworms. Treatment. **Rectal Splits and Fissures. Cystocoel and Rectocoel.** How to control rectocoel or cystocoel. When your doctor can give worthwhile help with rectocoel and cystocoel. **Cystitis.** Home care for early and mild cystitis. Spasm-soothing suppositories. How to ward off toilet paper cystitis. Honeymoon cystitis. Sex position during highly active periods. Drink plenty of water. When your doctor can give worthwhile help with cystitis. Bedwetting.

Female Troubles. Whitish discharge. How to control itching at the female opening. **Masturbation.** Reassurance. Masturbation injury. Undue sexual curiosity. **Common Male Sex Miseries.** Crab lice. Crotch itch. Penile irritations. Smegma irritation. Irritation after intercourse. Irritation from harsh chemicals. How to control urethritis. What about "morning pearl"? Prostate congestion. Prostate infection. Prostate disorder proneness. Prostate enlargement. Hot packs. **Menopause.** Fight menopausal blues with this philosophy. How to enjoy sex after the menopause. How to develop sexual skill.

Colds. Shorten colds with better drainage. Nose drops help shorten colds and make sinus infection less likely. Holding antibiotics in reserve. Controlled nose blowing.

Rest to build up your resistance. Aspirin. Dodge he-man germs during a cold. **Cold-Proneness.** Protect your nose lining against cold germs. Last-minute action to ward off a cold. Fight colds by mental measures. Build your cold-fighting morale. How to build cold-fighting morale. Have confidence in your body's powers. Other people's colds aren't easy to catch. Cold-fighting morale can really protect you. **Ordinary Sore Throat, Laryngitis, and Cough.** Hot gargles. Hot irrigations. Throat-soothing syrups. Laryngitis. Home measures for cough. Tight coughs. Loose cough. Rest. Fluids.

Nasal Crusting, Sore Nose, and Nosebleeds. Follow-up treatment. **Sinus Miseries, Stuffy Nose, Chronic Sore Throat, and Postnasal Drip.** Home care when sinus pain strikes. Aspirin. Nose drops or spray. Lightbulb baking. Hot applications. Nasal irrigation. Nasal siphonage. Stop using medicated nose drops, sprays, and jellies. Home decongestant method. Moisturizing spray. Restrain nose-blowing. Chin binder. Tunnel breathing and protective clothing. Antihistamines. Corrective measures against allergy. **Allergy.** Long-range relief from asthma, hay fever, and allergic sinus or rhinitis. Cold sores and fever blisters.

Headache. Home remedies for headache. Headaches from fatigue or tension. Rest in a darkened room. Hot towels. Fingertip massage. Postural headaches. Caffeine withdrawal headaches. Low blood sugar headaches. Migraine headaches. Eyestrain headaches. **Tooth Troubles.** How to relieve a toothache. Oil of cloves. Zinc-oxide-oil poultice. Abscessed teeth. Soft teeth. Home measures against periodontitis. Gum sores. Gum boils. **Danger Signals.** Pain in the eyes, over the eyes, or in the back of the head. Halos around lights. Abrupt worsening of vision. Eyes that thrive in gloom. A magenta band. **Eye Troubles.** How to remove a cinder from your eye. Tired eyes, TV eyes. Bloodshot or burning eyes, including pink-eye. Sties. **Common Ear Problems.** Ear drops. How to keep ear wax from piling up. Boils in the ear canals. Itching or discomfort in the ear canals.

Skin Irritations and Allergies. Sensitive skin. Weeping or blistered skin. Soothing soaks. Skin-healing baths. Colloid baths. Soothing measures for red or raw skin eruptions. Lotion. Pastes and ointments. Home correctives for common skin sensitivities. Specific skin irritations. Soap-burnt hands. Itching scalp. Laundry detergent rash. Cosmetic rash. Workman's eruption. Rash from medicines. **Skin Infections.** Boils, ingrown hair, and infected sores. Infection around a fingernail. How to cure athlete's foot with home measures. Sock sterilization. Psoriasis. The itch. Head lice, body lice, crab lice and bedbugs. **Leisure Time Skin Assaults.** Bee sting. Mosquito and other insect bites. Poison ivy. Sunburn. **Blackheads and Pimples.**

Bruises, Strains, and Sprains. How to make sure that you don't have a fracture. How to hold down damage. How to speed recovery. Stubbed small toe. Sprained big toe. Arch strain. Strained or sprained ankle. Strained or sprained thumb. Strained or sprained finger. Baseball fingers. Strained or sprained wrist. Persistent discomfort in sprains or strains. Blown-up knee or elbow bursa. Other bruising or wrenching injuries. Mashed fingers or toes. Sprained knees. Healing sprains and trick knees. How to cure back sprains and strains. How to prevent recurrent back injuries. When your doctor can give worthwhile aid with backache and back injury. **Cuts, Scrapes, and Burns.** How to clean out a cut or scrape. How to use antiseptics. How to improve circulation in the healing sore. How to bandage a cut or scrape. The instant freeze for burns. Flame burns. Scalds and other non-flame burns. Frostbite. Splinters. Splinters under a fingernail. Gouged-out wounds.

Tension and Fatigue. Part by part relaxation. Insomnia-combatting relaxation. The tension-easing refresher slouch. Tranquilizing tubs. Wet sheet packs. Soothing massage. Lethargy-fighting tonics. Home saunas. How to tone up flabby muscles and do-nothing nerves with a sheet bath. Sex as a tonic. Don't let temporary sexual impairments add to your worries or depression. Tone up for sex when you suffer depression or jitters. **Frequent Fatiguing Disorders.** How to conquer ordinary low-grade anemia. Iron tablets. Overweight. Appetite-spoiling snacks. Reduction-aiding surrender. High water intake. Weight-aiding schedule. Underweight. Fatigue from testicular congestion. Fatigue from sexual over-indulgence. Types of fatigue for which your doctor's help is worthwhile. Blood loss anemia. Pernicious anemia. How to conquer fatigue due to a sluggish thyroid. How to conquer fatigue from overactive thyroid. How to avoid diabetes. How to hold diabetes in check.

Varicose Veins. How to tell if you have varicose veins. Home measures can stop the formation or growth of varicose veins. How to control varicose vein miseries. Gravity-aided vein flushing. Elastic bandages. Home treatment for varicose veins even if you think they aren't hurting you. When your doctor can give worthwhile help for varicose veins. **Phlebitis.** How to prevent fireman's phlebitis. How to dodge the phlebitis of immobility. How to interrupt migratory phlebitis. How to ward off infectious phlebitis. How to spot phlebitis before serious complications occur. **Dizzy Spells.** What to do. Balance organ dizziness. Overbreathing-type dizziness. How to manage fainting type dizziness. Posture change dizziness. Low blood-sugar dizziness. Dizziness from medicines. When your doctor can give worthwhile help for dizzy spells. **Cold Hands and Feet and Blood-Lack Leg Cramps.** Hot towels to the adjacent trunk area. Warm flannel.

Smoking and circulation. How to boost your circulation with home exercises. How Dave Porter improved his waning circulation. Further aids to circulation.

Heart Attack. Painful attacks can best be fought flat, right where they occur. Rest and calm. Smothering type heart attacks. A lazy, chair-borne ride. Rescue squad. **Heart and Artery Trouble.** Half of heart complaints not heart trouble. Stop heart failure before it starts. Twinges of heart misery give valuable warning. Sluggish heart action. Rheumatic fever. Penicillin or sulfa. **Chest Pains.** Gas pains. **Hardening of the Arteries.** Hardening of the arteries controllable. Why cholesterol forms scales within artery walls. Attacks on the artery-hardening mechanism. Fat determines cholesterol in blood. Grocer's shelf foods for supple arteries. Keep down harmful fat with your meat. Use *liquid* cooking oils. Keep down total fuel value of foods. An artery-preserving diet tasty, varied, easy to follow. Artery-sparing diets may soon be unnecessary. **Coronary Heart Trouble.** Open coronary arteries with muscular activity. Develop outlets for pent-up emotion. **How to Hold Down Blood Pressure.** Dodging excess salt. Self-assertion. Getting reassurance.

Avoiding many cancers. **Cancer-Spurring Irritation.** Cancer-causing ultraviolet rays. Protecting lungs against dangerous fumes and irritants. What about tobacco? **How to Quit Smoking.** Breathing exercises really work. Cleansing intimate body parts. **Helping Doctor Fight Cancer-Spurring Irritation.** Doctors cure cancer-spurring states at mouth of womb. Dentists help dodge cancer. **Growths and Cancer Vanguards.** Warts. Ganglion. How to pop a ganglion. Skin tags. **Cancer Vanguards.** Heaped-up skin cells. White patches. Moles. **Tumor Threats.** Doctors find cancer vanguards you'd never see. Doctors cure many cancers completely. A sore or spot that does not heal. A lump, bunch, or bulge. Breast examination. Unusual bleeding.

Unusual flux or discharge. Lasting stomach trouble. Change in your bowel habits. Change in voice or altered cough.

When You <u>Want</u> Children. Rhythm in reverse. Acid-fighting douches. Knee chest position. Some Children But Not Too Many. No Pregnancies, Please! Abstinence. Rhythm Methods. Douches. Sperm barriers. Coils and loops. Pregnancy pretense pills. How to prevent leg-vein clots with the pill. Cycle-confusing pills. Surgery. Birth Control Roundup.

Discomforts of Early Pregnancy. Constant Tiredness. Need for extra protein. Salt and fluid intake. Psychologic factors to consider. Morning sickness. Middle Month Miseries. Backache. Kidney infection. Leg cramps. Faintness when lying on your back. Obstetrical Emergencies. Early bleeding. Bleeding Emergencies. Steady pain. How to know labor pains as true or false. Ride to the Hospital. Pregnancy and Medication.

CHAPTER ONE

Home Remedies for Muscular Backache, Muscle Miseries and Foot Troubles

There's one time when our sturdy Minnesotans are not too proud of their strength and hardihood: when those bulging muscles begin to hurt. With almost forty inches of snow to shovel each year, muscular backaches sometimes seem to be the Gopher State's pet affliction. Even the happy exertions of a canoe trip through wilderness or a long hike through the color riot of the autumn forest sometimes impose later punishment in the form of stiff leg muscles or aching feet. Our hardy folk have learned to get to work on these discomforts right away with home measures, which usually bring quick relief.

HOME MEASURES AGAINST MUSCULAR BACKACHE

You can take effective steps right in your own home to relieve backache and keep it from troubling you further. The equipment you need costs very little, but will often give you complete relief. Here are specific directions:

Hot showers with Figure 8 movement. When your back begins to hurt after a session of difficult lifting and bending, you should start toward relief right away. A hot shower in the proper position will work wonders. Stand with both knees slightly bent and both hands on your thighs just above the knee. Rest a good bit of your weight on your arms to relieve your tired back of the burden. Let a needle spray of hot water play on the sore area. Now pretend that you are drawing tiny figure 8's in the air with the lower end of your spine. Raise and push back one hip slightly, raise and push back the other hip, return to normal position, lower and tuck in one hip, lower and tuck in the other. Repeat slowly for about ten minutes.

Your youngsters can use this same approach to avoid backache and stiffness after contact sports. I've actually seen several of the

University of Minnesota's Golden Gopher football teams going through this routine on the trainer's orders after a tough game or a trying workout. When your youngsters get into slam-bang athletics, show them this passage anu let them give special showers a try.

Aspirin. If the backache develops in spite of this maneuver, take aspirin after each meal and at bedtime for at least two days, two tablets at a dose if you weigh 150 pounds or less, three if you weigh more than 150. Continue half doses after pain subsides as long as you have any back discomfort whatever. Youngsters below age twelve usually heal faster without aspirin than with it, probably because they go back to full activity as soon as you relieve their discomfort.

Extra sleep support. You will get a lot of relief from sleeping on a firm bed. Sag-free sleeping lets your weight stretch tight muscles when sleep relaxes them, and definitely helps you to get well. A piece of one-inch plywood underneath a cotton mattress prevents sag. Put this arrangement on top of box or coil springs for firm but yielding support.

Paraffin baths. Paraffin gives at least as much benefit as expensive tissue-heating machine treatments which many patients take for back trouble. Paraffin baths are safe and inexpensive. You can learn the technique in five minutes, and re-use the same materials for weeks or months. Here are the details:

> Get the following materials together:
>> 1-2 lbs. paraffin, of the type sold in grocery and drug stores for sealing preserves.
>> Mineral oil.
>> Double boiler.
>> Dry towels.
>> Paint brush, with rubber-set bristles.

Melt the paraffin in the double boiler. Add 2 tablespoonfuls of mineral oil for each pound of paraffin. Let the mixture cool until a definite scum forms on the top. Break the scum and test further by putting in a half-inch square of paraffin, which should not melt when the temperature is right. Oil or shave the back if it is very hairy. Have a member of your family paint your back with the paraffin. After the first layer is firm, paint on another. Continue until paraffin is about ¼ inch thick. Cover with a dry towel to hold the heat. After thirty to forty-five minutes, remove the towel and peel off the paraffin-oil mixture. You will find that it comes off very easily. Save it, and use the same mixture over and over again. Add further oil to make later applications cooler, or add pure paraffin to make peeling easier if you will tolerate slightly higher temperatures.

After you get accustomed to the heat and the procedure, you may want to use pure paraffin instead of paraffin-oil mixture. Pure paraffin gives maximum heat and maximum benefit.

Massage. You can get a great deal of relief from backache with properly done massage. This treatment is especially effective if it follows immediately after a paraffin bath. Here's the technique:

> Strip and lie on your abdomen on a comfortable but firm surface. Get your helper to start with rhythmic top-to-bottom strokes along the muscle masses beside the spine. He can lubricate the skin with mineral oil or with liniment made from one part methyl salicylate (oil of wintergreen) and two parts camphor and soap liniment. After about five minutes of gentle stroking, when the tight back muscles begin to loosen up and relax somewhat, a kneading type of massage may prove helpful. This begins at the upper back. Your helper presses his fingers firmly (but not uncomfortably) into the muscle mass beside the spine. Continuing pressure, he moves them up and down as far as the elasticity of the skin permits. Then he slides the fingers down about one inch and repeats the kneading motion. He continues in this fashion down the length of the spine, and repeats the procedure for about five minutes. He should then go back to gentle stroking and taper the pressure and rhythm to a soothing conclusion for the massage. If you used mineral oil for lubrication, clean it off with rubbing alcohol. If you use the liniment, you will find that it soaks in.

How to conquer a tendency toward backache. You can prevent recurrence of most muscular backaches with simple home exercises. The muscles of your abdomen work through the leverage of your rib cage and pelvis to brace your back. The heavy muscles near the spine also do their part. Extra strength in these muscle groups makes a natural girdle which supports your spine from every angle, thus preventing most muscular backache and many more serious back injuries.

After a bout with backache, wait until your back is fairly comfortable, then strengthen your back-bracing muscles with these exercises:

1. Strengthen the back muscles by back arching. Lie on your abdomen on a rug or pad with your hands on the floor above your head and your legs straight. Lift your hands and your knees from the floor. Hold them up for three to five seconds. Relax for three to five seconds. Repeat five times.

2. Strengthen abdominal muscles with leg straightening. Lie on your back with your knees drawn up and your hands beside your hips. Slowly straighten your legs, keeping your feet about six inches above the floor. If the strain on the abdominal muscles becomes too great, do not try to straighten your legs all the way at first. When you have straightened them as far as is comfortable, slowly fold them again. Repeat five times.

3. For further abdominal strengthening, spread your arms straight

to the sides while lying on your back. Stretch out your legs with your feet about twelve inches apart. Slowly lift your right leg until it is perpendicular, and bring your foot across to touch the floor high up beside your left hip. Return your right leg by reversing the motions, and follow the same pattern with your left leg. Repeat five times.

For best results, you should do these exercises once or twice a day for three weeks. After you have built muscle strength, you can usually maintain it by doing exercises twice a week. Some people prefer to maintain strength with a sporting activity which exercises the trunk muscles, like bowling, swimming or golf. Do not try to accomplish the initial buildup with sports, though: home exercises work much better.

HOME MEASURES FOR MUSCULAR MISERIES, CRAMPS, AND CHARLEY HORSES

When you overdo, your muscles usually give you plenty of misery. Most people sweat out this kind of discomfort because they can't afford to doctor for it. There is a lot of relief with these home techniques, though:

How to relieve aching muscles. At the first sign of muscular aching after any unusual work or muscle strain, start a three-pronged attack on muscle miseries:

Take aspirin. Start with two tablets after each meal and at bedtime if you weigh less than 150 pounds, three tablets at a dose if you weigh 150 pounds or more. Continue for at least two days, whether you think you need it or not. Then take half doses until the misery is completely gone.

Apply heat. A tub bath with moderately hot water, between 98 and 108 degrees, may be very helpful for general aching. If only one or two muscles are sore, you may get relief with hot towels, folded until six to eight layers thick, dipped in water at about 112 degrees, and covered with a dry towel to help hold the heat. Hot towels are more helpful if they are applied somewhat toward the heart from the sore area as well as directly over it: treat a sore forearm with hot towels wrapped nearly to the shoulder, for instance.

Improve blood drainage. A very substantial portion of muscular aching is due to accumulated chemical wastes. You can relieve this condition with circulation-aiding massage and downhill drainage. The aching extremity should be arranged on pillows so that it is several inches above the level of your chest. Slow massage is very helpful, using limp fingers, rhythmic strokes and mineral oil for lubrication. Each stroke of the massage should start at the most distant point from the heart and run up the affected extremity. After ten minutes or so of gentle stroking, a somewhat deeper pressure with the palm of the hand often helps, milking body juices from the sore area toward the heart. Five minutes or so of such milking, followed by a gradual taper to very gentle massage again, gives a great deal of relief and definitely speeds healing. Clean off the mineral oil with rubbing alcohol. Repeat the procedure once or twice a day until the aching subsides.

Neck and shoulder-arm pain. Years ago at Minnesota's Mayo Clinic, one of my doctor friends found his office filled with a steady succession of hard-working farm and laboring people with neck and shoulder-arm pain. He knew that this pain often stemmed from one of life's great vicious circles: muscular discomfort leading to muscle spasm which in turn pinches nerves and leads to further discomfort. Time after time, my friend relieved victims of persistent or recurrent miseries by stretching over-tight muscles. The key step, he found, was stretching the muscles around the spinal column in the neck and upper back. At first, he did this with a special leather head halter and a complicated arrangement of pulleys and weights. As the years went by, however, my friend saw that many poor workers had to stay away from their homes for weeks at a time and many good Minnesota farmers had to trek miles several times each week to take full advantage of this treatment. He devised a simple home method which they now apply right in their own homes to get the same relief clinic treatment once afforded.

You can often get a great deal of help with any kind of muscular or arthritic discomfort in the neck, upper back, or shoulder and arm with home-fashioned means of neck stretching. If you can't afford to buy a head sling from the nearest surgical supply house, you can make one out of table felt from any dry goods store. Start with a double thickness two inches wide and two yards long. Sew the ends together solidly to make a single loop. Put your head through the middle of this loop and hold the ends of it with one hand in the vicinity of each shoulder. Twist the ends you have in your hands half a turn, so that the loop crosses itself at each side of your neck. Raise the two ends up above your head, keeping the center portion of the loop tucked under your chin in the front and beneath the curve of your head in the back. At the point where the strips cross above your ears, pin with two safety pins. Adjust so that the head sling will slip on and off easily and so that the side loops are approximately equal in length. Replace the pins with firm stitching if you wish.

Whether you buy or make your head sling, you will need to suspend a sturdy wooden coathanger directly over your head. A hook screwed into a door frame or other support works very well to hold the coathanger. After adjusting the sling at your chin and the nape of your neck, put the side loops or traction straps of the sling across the coathanger arms. Bend your knees slightly so that your body weight produces steady muscle-stretching action all along the upper spine. Adjust the sling so that your head remains upright instead of tipping backward during the stretch, and settle down for a steady five to ten minute spasm soothing session. Some of my Minnesota angler patients put a spring type fish scale between the coathanger and the supporting hook or eyelet to help them determine how much to bend their knees. Ten to 15 pounds is the limit with recent or extreme neck pain. Victims of smoldering, long-lasting miseries sometimes must work gradually up to 50 pounds.

Muscle cramps. Gentle kneading, preferably through several layers of warm, wet towel or with the part immersed in warm water, gives quick relief from ordinary muscle cramps. The towels or water should be lukewarm, not hot (about 98 degrees). Start kneading somewhat below the cramped muscle, keeping your fingers together and using their flat surfaces instead of their tips. Knead upward toward the trunk as if you were working oleomargarine in a plastic bag. Repeat several times with gradually deeper kneading. A warm flannel wrap helps to keep down later soreness.

If you get muscle cramps mainly from swimming or unusual exertion, you can usually control your tendency toward them by taking several simple precautions:

Extra salt. Exertion causes sweating. Sweat carries salt out of your body. Unless you take enough salt to replace what you lose, muscle fibers become irritable from the low salt level in tissue fluids around them. This muscle irritability is the cause of most cramps at work, in the swimming pools, and at sporting events. Big time football players dodge this problem by drinking a solution of half a teaspoonful of salt to each glass of water whenever they practice or play. You can use the same approach, or you can take heat fatigue type salt tablets if you prefer—one tablet for each extra glass of water you drink.

Vein flushing exercises. Leg cramps that come on after you have been standing a great deal usually are due to accumulation of chemical wastes in the muscles. Your leg veins do not flush chemical wastes out of your muscles very effectively when you are standing, especially if you have any varicose veins. The best way to keep from getting leg cramps is to take time out every two hours when you are on your feet to do this exercise: Take off your shoes and socks. Lie on your back with hips raised on a pillow or on the arm of an overstuffed davenport or chair. Put your feet high in the air, and jiggle them rapidly with the ankles and toes completely relaxed for a period of 30 seconds.

Bed cradles. Muscle cramps during the night often stop if you keep the weight of covers off your feet. Trim two ordinary cardboard cartons from the grocery store down to an upright rectangle of cardboard for the bottom of the bed, a bracing triangle at each side, and a steadying base to tuck under the mattress. Put these cardboard corners in place over the bottom sheet and underneath the other covers. If you find the extra comfort you obtain with supported bedclothing is worthwhile, you may want to buy a metal bed cradle from your druggist or surgical supply house.

Quinine. If night cramps persist in spite of support for bed-clothing, take one quinine tablet (five grains) each day for ten days. This usually gives at least six months relief. Quinine is perfectly safe in this dosage unless you are pregnant or have disease of the arteries, in which case you should check with your doctor first. You should time dosage to avoid menstrual periods.

Charley horses. A Charley horse is a muscle cramp which is so severe that it wrenches some muscle fibers loose and causes bleeding into the muscle itself. The blood which leaks out between muscle fibers causes irritation and further muscle spasm.

Cold. Immediate first aid for a Charley horse aims at shrinking blood vessels to limit internal bleeding. An ice pack is the best measure, and should be available at athletic contests and other places where muscle strain is expected.

Heat. You can safely use heat after only a few minutes in treating a Charley horse. Muscle tissue contains a special substance which makes blood vessels seal themselves off almost instantly, so that further seepage of the kind which makes bruises extend themselves does not occur. Hot towels or hot soaks give considerable relief.

Other measures. Contrast baths, as described under "Painful Arches" on page 30, help if soreness persists. Gentle kneading massage for ten minutes after heat treatment may help to speed healing, too.

HOME CARE FOR FOOT TROUBLES

Almost everyone suffers at times from corns and callouses, blisters, and ingrown toenails, aching arches, or tired feet. Foot miseries are big miseries. If your feet hurt, you hurt all over. If your feet are tired, you are tired all over. Here's what to do for immediate relief and for permanent, lifelong cure of most common foot troubles:

How to trim corns and callouses. You can trim your own corns and callouses safely, unless you have diabetes or disease of the arteries. Wash your feet thoroughly and soak them in warm water for twenty minutes. Soak a new single-edged razor blade in rubbing alcohol, and use the same disinfectant to clean the corn or callous and the nearby skin. Wash your hands. Trim from the edge of the corn or callous toward the center, your blade almost parallel to the skin. Quit if you draw blood. Check with your doctor if you can't trim what seems to be a callous without drawing blood: you may have a wart which needs special treatment.

Relieve pressure to rid yourself of corns and callouses. Pressure, not rubbing, actually causes most corns and callouses. You can actually rid yourself of corns and callouses by properly fitted shoes, possibly with some felt pads. Properly fitted shoes also reduce foot strain and take much of the ache out of sagging arches. In checking my own patients, I've found about one in five grossly misfitted. The only way to be sure your shoes are right for you is to double check the fit yourself. Here's how to do it:

1. Check length by feeling for the ball of your foot, not the end of your toes. Feel along the side of the shoe and locate the knob at the base of your big toe, which should be just at the sharpest-curving point on the inside edge of your shoe sole. Always check standing as well as sitting because your feet may spread half a size or more under the burden of your body weight. Fit the longer foot, if they are different.

2. Check width. Feel for fit across the front of your foot and your little toe, with at least part of your weight on the foot. Pressure, not rubbing, causes blisters, corns, and callouses. Be sure you have enough room for your little toe when your weight is on your foot.

3. Check the shoes for bight. When you roll your weight up on the front part of your foot at the beginning of each step, creases in the leather may pinch you. Spot this while you're still in the store, and have the salesman put in a bight block to prevent it.

4. See whether the heel fits snugly, or whether it slips up and down easily. If you can't get shoes that fit both the front and the back of your foot properly, fit the front of your foot and get the heel padded or taken in. Most good shoe stores will fit a butterfly-shaped felt pad into your heels at no extra charge, with one wing on each side and a narrow strip around the back. Or you can get a shoemaker to take in the heel or fit molded heel counters, either of which should cost about one dollar.

Felt pads. If perfectly fitted shoes still leave slight pressure or friction at certain spots on your foot or if bony prominences push out against the skin, padding may be the only answer. However, *the object of padding is to spread weight or pressure to other parts of the foot or other parts of the affected bone, not to cushion the sore spot itself.* A thin layer of table felt cemented to the side and top of your shoe to hold the outer edge of your foot away from the leather may help corns. Some patients find that a sleeve of felt about four inches wide around the foot from the ankle to the base of the toes takes the weight off of callouses at the front of the foot and holds the leather away from corns simultaneously. If your toes curl sharply or if the end of one or more foot bones carries an undue share of weight so that it pushes against the skin from inside, a special type of felt pad called a metatarsal bar may help. A metatarsal bar attaches to the inside of your sole near the front of your arch. It cures corns by shifting the position of the toes on the ends of the foot bones so that they stay straight instead of curling. It cures callouses by spreading the weight across all four small foot bones instead of letting too much of it rest on one or two bone ends. Many shoe and drug stores sell metatarsal bars in three thicknesses and several sizes. Try medium thickness first. Determine where to place them in your shoes by laying a lead pencil on its side and stepping on it barefooted. Try first with the pencil about one inch behind the front of your arch, at the same angle as the bases of your four smaller toes. Find the exact space and angle at which your toes curl the least and your feet feel most comfortable. Then glue the metatarsal bars to the corresponding spot in your shoes.

Relief from blisters. If new shoes or unusual exertions give you blisters on the hands or feet, adhesive tape bracing usually gives prompt relief. Wash the blistered part thoroughly with soap and water. Let it dry. Cut several four-inch strips of inch-wide cloth adhesive tape. Apply the center of one strip to the blister with at least ¼ inch of its upper margin on normal skin and smooth the ends into contact with the skin. Apply other overlapping strips until the entire blister and a margin of normal skin is smoothly covered with tape. Leave this in place for five days, then remove. The dead surface layer of the blister usually hangs limp by this time. You can trim it off with scissors or let it dry.

If the blister bursts before you get a chance to apply tape, or if it is larger than half a dollar, you can wash the area thoroughly, trim off the blister's roof, and keep a bandage lined with Telfa or a mild antiseptic ointment in place over it for four or five days.

Relief for painful arches. You can get a lot of relief from arch discomfort with "contrast baths." Fill one bucket or basin with moderately hot water, another with moderately cold. Ideal temperatures are 105 degrees and 50 degrees, but these need not be exact. Soak the affected part in hot water for four minutes, in cold for one minute, then back into the hot. Alternate for about thirty minutes. Always begin and end with the hot soak.

Massage also helps painful feet, especially if it is done immediately after a contrast bath. The object of the massage is to milk strain-produced chemical wastes out of the feet and ankles, not to rub the sore ligaments and muscles. You should lie down with your legs comfortably arranged on two or more pillows. Dry the legs thoroughly and powder them well with talc. If you have a helper, ask him to make a collapsible ring by joining the tips of his thumbs and forefingers. Starting at the base of the toes, he should draw this finger-thumb ring up the length of the foot and lower leg, milking blood and tissue fluid toward the heart. Repeat rhythmically with gradually increasing pressure for five to ten minutes, tapering off to gentle pressure before ending the massage. If you have no one to help you, you can lie on your back with one or two pillows under your hips and your legs drawn up. In this position you can perform massage for yourself without fighting the pull of gravity on body fluids, although you may find this rather tiring.

Adolescent arch strain. After either an athletic event or a day which involves unusual amounts of standing and walking, teenagers and young adults sometimes get pain along the inner and lower margins of the arch. There may be slight swelling and tenderness in this area, but there should not be tenderness at any spot along the bones of the top of the foot. Bony tenderness sometimes points toward so-called "march fractures"—tiny cracks in the bones which occur with prolonged hiking, especially over rough ground—and these require a doctor's care. Otherwise, arch pain usually responds to home measures.

Contrast baths, as described in the last paragraph, give some immediate relief. In some instances, a well-fitting hunter's boot or other firm, solid-soled shoe will give enough support. It is best to wear such shoes all the time rather than go barefoot or switch to soft slippers, since the shoe's sole acts as a splint. If these measures do not control discomfort, the foot will have to be strapped with adhesive tape.

Tricks for taping. Try to avoid waterproof tape if possible—it traps sweat underneath and peels off more quickly. Shave off any long hairs, which will otherwise cause discomfort when the tape is removed. The tape will stick better and cause less irritation if you paint the skin underneath with tincture of benzoin (available at any drugstore without prescription). Let this coat dry thoroughly before beginning the tape job.

There are several tricks you can use to apply adhesive tape smoothly to any body part. Measure the approximate length of a strip by unrolling it and laying the back of the tape (not the sticky side) against the skin. At the same time, you can check the way the tape will follow body contours, making it easier to wind up the right place when you apply it "for keeps." Cut several strips at a time and apply them from the middle rather than from one end, smoothing the tape into place without pulling or stretching it, with the direction determined entirely by body contours. Overlap strips by 1/3 their width—narrow gaps between strips, which sometimes occur when you cut your margins too close, cut painfully with the least swelling. If it is practical, apply an elastic bandage over your tape job for a few hours at least—tape sticks much better if it is kept in close contact with the skin until it is thoroughly warm.

Tape for arch strain. Use 1-inch tape cut to lengths of 15 to 18 inches. Have the patient turn his or her foot outward (toward the little toe side) as far as possible. Angle the middle of one piece of tape across the inner side of the heel and smooth it into contact with the skin in both directions. One end should wind up on the top of the arch, coming up from its outer rim. The other should come around the outside of the ankle and end at or near the junction of the top of the foot and the ankle. Place three or four additional strips parallel to the first, overlapping about 1/3 of the tape width.

Now have the patient turn the foot inward as far as possible. The tape already applied should hold the heel in an outward-rolled position, so that this movement should have the effect of increasing the height of the arch and relieving strain on its ligaments. Start the middle of a piece of tape along the bottom of the foot near the bases of the toes. The ends should follow the foot contours in a spiral up the arch, joining (at some rather unpredictable point) the tape already applied to the heel. Apply three or four further overlapping strips behind the first. It is more important to keep the tape smooth and apply it without pull than it is to get it to go in the right direction. To finish covering the entire foot, use either a spiral of tape or a series of encircling strips around the arch, applied smoothly and without tension.

This tape should be left in place for a week or ten days, or reapplied in the same fashion if it becomes either loose or intolerably dirty.

Long-range help with arch troubles. If you have painful or weak arches, here's a step-by-step approach to your long-range problem:

1. Get oxford-type shoes that fit your arch properly by following the four steps outlined above.

2. If you still have discomfort, get cork shoe inserts to prop up the crucial parts of your arch. Do these two foot exercises daily for three weeks:

> Pick up one dozen ¾ inch marbles with the toes of each foot, and deposit them in a hat or box.
>
> Stand on your toes in your bare feet. Turn your ankles about halfway inward. Roll your weight slowly down along the outside of your feet until it rests on your heels. Repeat ten times.

3. If this gives relief most of the time, control occasional discomfort after special strain with contrast baths (detailed directions on page 30).

4. If you continue to have trouble and are over age forty, get rigid plastic or steel and leather arch supports. Such supports give comfort at the price of weakening your foot muscles and making your need for arch supports likely to increase. But they *do* give comfort, which makes them worthwhile when other measures have failed.

Bunions. When the ball of your foot splays out at the base of your big toe, pressure against the side of your shoe often causes swelling and pain. You can usually get relief from such discomfort with contrast baths and aspirin. To keep the bunions from getting worse and ultimately requiring operation, these further steps are worthwhile:

1. Get at least one pair of low heeled lacing oxfords for everyday wear, and have your shoemaker attach an anterior heel, which is a block of leather toward the front of the arch which spreads your

weight to the foot bones instead of letting it roll up on the ball of your foot with each stride.

2. Stick to low or medium heels even for dress-up occasions. High heels more than double the weight on the front part of the foot, which definitely makes bunions worse.

Ingrown toenail. Home care usually relieves ingrown toenail temporarily, and sometimes gives a permanent cure. If a deep spur, severe infection, or some health problem like diabetes complicates the problem, best see your doctor right away. Otherwise try these home measures:

1. Hot soaks. The corner of your nail usually digs in enough to cause redness, swelling and pain before you realize that anything is wrong. Hot soaks for 20 minutes three or four times a day help to take the redness and swelling out.

2. Side and center trimming. As soon as hot soaks have settled down the tenderness to allow relatively pain-free handling, you want to remove the corner of the toenail which is digging into your flesh. While the nail is still soft after a soak, clean the toe with alcohol. Wash your hands thoroughly. Rest the toe against a firm surface like the top of a footstool or low table. Peel the fold of skin off the base of the nail with an orange stick or the end of a fingernail file. With a clean, new, single edged razor blade, make a cut part way through the nail, beginning at the side of the nail just above its base and cutting straight toward the tip of the toe. Start far enough down to leave a long, smooth incline which will push the skin back as the nail grows out. Deepen this cut until the fragment of nail which has dug in is nearly free. With manicure scissors and tweezers, free up the loose portion and remove it. In the same way, remove a narrow pie-shaped wedge from the center of the nail with its base at the nail end and its point about half way up the nail. This makes the edge of the nail more yielding and improves your chance of getting the nail corner to grow out past the skin instead of digging in. As the nail grows out, soak the toe and recut this pie-shaped wedge at intervals.

3. Petroleum jelly corner-lifting packs. You can keep the advancing corner of the nail from digging in by pushing a small piece of petroleum jelly impregnated gauze underneath it daily. Unravel a roll of one inch roller gauze into a wide mouthed jar. Add about one ounce of petroleum jelly. Heat uncovered in a warm oven for thirty minutes. The melted petroleum jelly will impregnate the gauze. For use, cut off a small piece of the gauze and pack it under the advancing corner of the toenail with a toothpick or small finishing nail. The petroleum jelly keeps the nail more yielding, and the packing helps lift it out of the flesh.

4. Get shoes with extra toe room. If you have ever had ingrown nails, you need shoes with a straight inner margin instead of pointed toes, and preferably with a box or a moccasin type front.

CHAPTER TWO

Home Remedies for Arthritis and Rheumatism

If Minnesotans weren't so blasted stoical, they would eat aspirin by the ton for creaking joints. The hard physical work of farming and forestry plus plenty of he-man outdoor recreation puts lots of strain on North Country spines and joints. We have more than our share of arthritics here. My patients have had more than enough chance to try various home remedies and correctives for arthritis, aching joints, bursitis and other forms of rheumatism. Here are the measures they've found most effective through the years:

HOME MEASURES FOR JOINT PAINS

Whether you suffer from stiff fingers, painful joints, or full-blown arthritic disease, joint trouble gives you real misery. Probably the more severe forms of arthritis will drive you to your doctor, whose new hormone-type treatments and other measures give definite protection from crippling and, often give superior relief. You might get enough extra relief from Indocin, which needs a doctor's supervision because of occasional harmful effects on your blood, to make prescription care worthwhile. New muscle relaxants are also "prescription only," and help if muscle spasms or motion-limiting muscle stiffness contributes to your miseries. But home measures usually help whether you are taking prescription medicines or not.

Red, swollen joints. Active joint disease with swelling, redness, heat and pain calls for gentle, soothing measures. Intense heat, massage, or exercise merely adds to the congestion and makes the situation worse. At this stage, these techniques usually prove most helpful:

The hormone stimulating aspirin dose. Doctors have known for years that aspirin relieves joint and muscle aches much more completely if you take it according to a certain dosage pattern: high doses the first day or two, with smaller but still regular doses thereafter. Recently they found out why this is true. Used in high starting, steady doses, aspirin definitely spurs your body to form cortisone and its hormone cousins—the great new miracle drugs that have put even crippled, bedridden victims of arthritis back on their feet! You can get the benefit of medicine's best and most costly treatment for your joint and muscle aches simply by taking aspirin according to this plan:

> As long as you are an adult, take aspirin tablets on arising, after breakfast, lunch, and supper, and at bedtime. The number of tablets at each dose depends upon your weight. If you weight 100-135 pounds, take 2 tablets at each dose for a total of ten tablets daily. If you weigh 136-170 pounds, take 3 tablets at each dose for a total of fifteen tablets daily. If you weigh over 170 pounds, take three tablets on arising and at bedtime and four tablets after each meal for a total of eighteen tablets daily.
>
> Continue this dosage for three days or until you feel considerably better. Then drop the morning dose, continuing the other four doses daily. Continue to take the tablets regularly, even if you need them over a period of years. If you think you need less medicine, take one less tablet for your evening dose, wait three days and if still feeling well cut another of your doses, and so on.

A lot of people worry about whether aspirin will subtly undermine their blood or general health when used over a period of months or years. The answer is, *absolutely no*, if you never take it on an empty stomach. Any harmful effects which have been reported stem from blood seepage within the stomach, caused by the irritating effect of undiluted aspirin lying directly against the stomach wall. Unless aspirin causes clear-cut distress, the program recommended above is entirely harmless. If you get heartburn or nausea after taking aspirin, take it after meals, drink milk instead of water with each pill, or switch to either buffered aspirin or coated tablets of sodium salicylate (which don't dissolve until they get through your stomach). If you still get nauseated, or if you get dizzy from aspirin, you're the one person in several thousand who is allergic to it and has to use other means of relief.

Red joints in children. Red, swollen joints often signal rheumatic fever rather than simple joint disease in children, adolescents and young adults. The larger joints—knees, ankles and elbows—are more likely than smaller ones to be involved. One joint will usually flare, then clear up in a day or two, with other joints flaring up in succession. Victims often have some fever, but may have normal temperature. Since rheumatic fever can present quite varied fronts in different cases and may involve the heart, it is always wise to get a doctor in on the case right away whenever you even suspect that this condition *might* be present.

Warm flannel. You can usually get some relief from swollen-joint pain with warm flannel wrappings. The easiest method is to wrap or cover the joint with two or three layers of flannel and cover loosely with a heating pad set for low heat. Remove or shift the pad as the flannel reaches a cozy warmth. Keep the joint lightly warmed for about an hour at a time, three or more times a day.

Diet. Two of the three common forms of joint trouble respond to shifts in diet. Rheumatoid arthritis, which usually starts in people who have not yet turned 40 and tends to leave stiffened joints in the wake of each attack, seems to improve somewhat on a *low residue diet.* Omit raw vegetables, cabbage, brussels sprouts, broccoli, and bran cereals. The commonest cause oɪ red, swollen joints which first give trouble after age 40 is gout. The main tip-off to the early stages of this condition is that the joints become severely inflamed, often in the middle of the night, but usually subside completely without residual stiffness after a few days or weeks. Gout often occurs in people who are not addicted to high living. It affects the joint at the base of the toe, which most people think is typical of the disease, less than one fifth of the time. A *low purine diet* helps a great deal. Omit organ meats like sweetbreads and liver, navy and similar type beans, and soups or gravies. If you suspect gout, or if these foods make your joint trouble worse, check with your doctor for a more thorough diet and for special medicines if required.

Bodily rest. You can build your recuperative powers to fight arthritis with extra rest. Several breaks during the day are always helpful. More complete bed rest usually helps if you have fever, weakness, or widespread involvement.

Rest for sore joints. Using red, swollen joints does much more harm than good, even though you definitely need the courage to use parts in spite of some discomfort when they are mildly involved or have begun to mend. If a joint becomes stiff and sore after a certain amount of use, or if it stiffens up 6 to 12 hours later, you should do somewhat less next time.

Motion preserving exercises. You can cut your chance of later stiffness or crippling quite substantially by carrying each swollen joint through its entire range of motion several times a day. Do this immediately after or toward the end of the warm flannel treatment. If the involved joint is a hinge, like a finger joint, elbow or knee, move it all the way one way then the other. More complex joints call for several varieties of loosening movement: you want to free up a sore shoulder so that you can raise your arm, move it forward and back, and rotate it, for instance.

Supported or flotation exercises. Some patients find that they do better with motion-preserving exercises if the weight of the moving part is supported. You can exercise under water in a warm tub, so that the part floats virtually weightless. You can support ailing parts with healthy ones, or get someone to help you. Do not force the part beyond where you can move it with its own muscles, though. Just relieve the burden imposed by the weight of the moving part.

Cripple-cutting braces. Even total loss of function in a joint usually involves very little crippling or disability if the joint freezes in a highly usable position. If you have a prolonged bout with joint trouble, make sure that the parts involved stay useful by bracing them in a workable position during your hours of rest. Follow these suggestions according to the parts involved:

Back: Sleep on a cotton mattress, bedboard and coil spring arrangement as described above on page 22. Sleep on your back with a small pillow or rolled blanket between your shoulder blades so that the weight of your shoulders will keep them square. Place sandbags (made at home from light canvas) along both sides of your body so that you will not roll over during the night. Place a small pillow under your neck if necessary for comfort, but never place a pillow under your head.

Hips: Keep the legs from rolling outward by laying sandbags along the outside of your thigh and leg. Your toes should point straight up when you are in bed.

Knees: Lay sandbags along the sides of your legs to keep them straight so that the weight of your leg straightens your knees. If any stiffness develops, your legs will then remain entirely usable. Arthritics who sleep with their legs bent or with pillows under their knees sometimes find themselves in a crippling half-stoop if joints freeze up even slightly.

Ankles, feet, and toes: A footboard saves lots of crippling here! Cut a board 18 inches wide, one inch thick and four inches shorter than the width of your bed. Nail short crosspieces at right angles extending toward the head of the bed, to fit beneath the mattress and hold the footboard in perpendicular position. Place the footboard inside the top sheet when you make the bed. Keep your feet against it as you sleep to hold your ankles at the proper right angle and keep the weight of the covers from twisting inflamed toes.

Shoulders: Sleep with a pillow or sandbag between your elbow and your body to assure proper spacing.

Elbows: Keep your elbows partly bent, either by placing sandbags under them and laying your hands across your body or by raising your hands and forearms on two pillows. Even a totally stiff elbow is no great handicap if you can still get your hand to your mouth and comb your hair.

Wrists If your hand is tipped up at the wrist, you can use your finger muscles much more strongly than if the wrist is bent. A leather-padded metal splint helps to hold your hand up during the night. Buy one from the nearest surgical supply house, or have your shoemaker make a brace which fits from your palm to your midforearm. As a temporary measure, you can wrap the hand and wrist with an elastic bandage each night. With the wrist tipped up and the bandage partially stretched, wrap alternate turns around the wrist and around the hand at the base of the fingers, crossing at the back of the wrist or hand.

Subsiding or smoldering joint trouble: Home treatment really comes into its own in smoldering or subsiding joint troubles. You can't always afford a doctor for dragged-out complaints, and these difficulties yield especially well to remedies you can manage for yourself. Use full hormone-spurring doses of aspirin without fear, and take these additional measures:

Sore, stiff fingers yield very well to paraffin dip baths. Melt and cool paraffin-oil mixture as described on page 22. After testing the temperature, dip your better hand quickly in the paraffin. As soon as the first layer is set, dip again. Repeat until the paraffin forms a glove ¼ inch or more in thickness. Wrap in a dry towel to hold the heat. Now dip your worse hand in the mixture several times, letting each layer set before dipping again. When the paraffin forms a ¼ inch glove, immerse the whole hand in the melted paraffin and hold it there. The soothing warmth will penetrate all the way through your fingers inside twenty to thirty minutes.

Aching arms, hips, or knees. Painted on paraffin does wonders here. Prepare the paraffin, then paint it on with a paint brush in layers until it is at least ¼ inch thick. Wrap with a dry towel to hold the heat. Peel off after thirty minutes, and follow with a rubdown using this homemade liniment:

Methyl salicylate (wintergreen)	¼ cup
Camphor and soap liniment	¾ cup

You can get these ingredients in any drug store, and mix them together in a clean, stoppered bottle. Shake well before each use. Rub in around the aching joint for 10 to 15 minutes.

Perpetual stiff neck. Make yourself a neck-stretching sling, as described on page 25. While your neck is under moderate stretch, turn your head far to the right. Place the heel of your right hand against the left side of your chin and gently press straight back. Repeat, turning your head to the left. Do this three times on each of three occasions through the day.

Stiff elbows, wrists, ankles, and toes. Use contrast baths for these forms of misery, following the directions on page 30. Paraffin baths help, too.

Diffuse joint trouble. When a patient tells me that he aches all over or points to half a dozen different ailing joints, I usually ask him to build himself a baker. The essential features are several light bulbs and sockets, a reflecting surface of metal or foil, and a frame which holds the light bulbs with the reflector about 18 inches away from the painful body parts. Most patients make a rod iron and sheet tin or aluminum structure in the shape of a tunnel (as one of the two parts of a cylinder cut in half along its length), then fasten two to four sockets to its under surface for a bank of 100- to 200-watt light bulbs. The heat from light bulbs in such a unit is very soothing and much more even than that you get from a heating pad or single-unit heat lamp. You can lie with your sore joints underneath the baker for 30 to 45 minutes once or twice each day.

Home whirlpool equipment. Although the equipment is rather expensive, several of my patients have reported worthwhile relief from home whirlpool treatments. A special pump swirls the water in your bathtub around and fills it with tiny air bubbles. The effect is of combined heat and massage, easily applied without assistance to almost any body part. The outfit my patients use is made by Jacuzzi Bros. Inc. here in Minneapolis, but there may be others just as good. I wouldn't try to improvise a homemade substitute because of the danger of electric equipment around bathroom fixtures. For red or swollen joints, only moderately warm water (about 108° F.) works best. Smoldering miseries may respond to somewhat warmer temperatures (about 112° F.).

Hip, knee, and joint strain. You can avoid or relieve a great deal of joint distress by controlling strain in weight bearing joints. These joints can usually bear up under their normal share of your normal weight. But an overloaded joint is like a tire on a car that's loaded until the wheels scrape the fenders. A little extra weight causes a lot of extra strain, wear, and tear.

Aching knees, for instance, are often due to extra strain produced when flat feet shift the muscle pulls in the leg. In other cases, undue strain on the knees stems from knock-knees or bow-legs. You can relieve most such undue strain in a hurry with inconspicuous shoe wedges that rebalance your weight. Here's the step-by-step program:

1. Get a pair of oxford style shoes, with at least four eyelets for laces on each side and with low heels.

2. Unless the heels fit so snugly that your feet will not roll inside the shoes even a fraction of an inch, get your shoemaker to make molded heel counters (cost: about $1.00).

3. Have half inch heel wedges put on for another dollar or less to tip your feet as follows: for flat feet or knock knees, have wedges installed on the *inside* of your heels, shifting extra weight to the outer, little-toe side of your foot. For bow legs, have wedges installed on the *outside* of your heels to shift extra weight to the arched side of your foot (but fit arch supports at the same time if your feet are the least bit weak—this position puts extra stress on the arches).

You can also relieve joint strain by shedding excess weight. Aching ankles, knees, and hips do better without the burden of extra pounds. Even a few pounds of weight loss often gives striking relief.

Growing pains. Minnesota brings out the vigor of the young. It's not just the great chances for outdoor activities—other places have toboggan slopes, ice rinks, and shovelable walks. It's the confounded cold, which keeps you going at full steam just to keep warm.

But youngsters in other regions aren't too much different. They race around at full speed, keep going until they're exhausted, and ignore the rough ground or poor footing. No wonder they get aches and pains occasionally! If you or I tried to keep up with one of them, we'd wind up sick in bed.

So they complain of muscle aches, joint pains, "stitches" (which are side aches caused by muscle spasm in the diaphragm), and so forth. Mainly your problem isn't what to do about these complaints—youngsters mend quickly, and the pains are often gone before you can get a boy or girl to hold still for warm soaks or swallow an aspirin. The problem is that "growing pains" sometimes turn out to be early evidence of rheumatic fever. Prompt identification and care for this disorder generally helps the victim to avoid heart involvement, so it pays to lean over backward in checking out any truly suspicious complaints.

The simplest checkup is still with the old thermometer. When a youngster complains of growing pains, your first step should be to take his temperature three times a day, in the morning, right after school and at bedtime. Shake the thermometer all the way down and be sure that it has registered completely (by reading it quickly, putting it back in the mouth for a while and reading it again until it stays the same). Sometimes you'll find a mildly elevated temperature in the afternoon when you hadn't noted fever. More important, you'll sometimes find a variation of more than one full degree between morning and evening readings. Even if none of the readings go over 98.6 degrees, more than a one degree low-high spread makes rheumatic fever a distinct possibility.

Finally, you can check for extra warmth or heat in the area of each complaint, especially if a joint is involved. Feel for temperature change with the back of your fingers or hand rather than with the palm (which is more sensitive to touch but less sensitive to warmth and cold). Compare the part that hurts with the opposite member, and if there is any trace of extra warmth arrange a further checkup with your doctor.

HOME REMEDIES FOR NEURITIS, BURSITIS, AND INFLAMED LEADER GUIDES

A great many of the miseries that go with rheumatism stem from other structures than the joints themselves. Some of these troubles come on with joint difficulty, others strike independently. Home measures help a great deal, with little or no expense.

Neuritis and neuralgia. If you tend toward joint trouble, you usually also suffer at times from shooting pains, numbness, tingling or supersensitive skin. Three measures help these complaints:

Vitamin B_1. Vitamin B_1 (thiamine) seems to speed healing of neuritis and neuralgia. Two 50 mgm. tablets a day is an average effective intake.

Massage with homemade wintergreen liniments. For this kind of discomfort, mix:

Methyl salicylate (oil of wintergreen)	½ cup
Camphor and soap liniment	½ cup

Rub in with long, even strokes for 10 to 15 minutes three times daily.

Flannel or cotton knit protection. The gentle softness and warmth of flannel wrapping or cotton knit long underwear proves very soothing to neuritis and neuralgia. Such dressing also prevents the discomfort caused by rubbing of harsher fabrics on raw-nerve sensitive skin.

Bursitis. Bursitis usually involves a shoulder, elbow, or knee. In these locations, muscles and tendons glide across each other or rub along bony prominences. Your body forms smooth-lined pockets of tissue to ease the. friction. When these bearing-sacs get sore, the scraping of raw, sensitive surfaces gives exquisite pain.

If you get severe bursitis, your doctor can give worthwhile help. Hydrocortisone injections, X-ray treatment and several other measures are very effective. With milder attacks, these four simple home remedies may do the trick:

Pressure bandaging. An elastic bandage wrapped snugly around the area involved often braces the inflamed bursa. You can usually wrap the area near a joint comfortably with Figure 8 loops—a turn above the joint, a diagonal turn down across it, a turn below the joint and a diagonal back up. Keep the bandage partly stretched as you apply it. If the bursa is very tender, wind on several strips of soft flannel before using the elastic bandage.

Lightbulb heat. Since the area involved in bursitis is usually fairly small, lightbulb heat from an ordinary desk lamp usually gives considerable relief. Place the bulb 12 to 18 inches from your bared skin. If you do not have a desk lamp or metal reflector, line a cloth shade with aluminum foil to help reflect and concentrate the heat.

Hormone-boosting doses of aspirin. For quick relief from bursitis, take aspirin in the dosage and with the precautions described on page 36. Continue half doses for at least a week after the disorder begins to subside.

Rest. Occasionally, the only way to get relief from bursitis is to keep from using the affected part for a few days. If an arm or shoulder is involved, a sling usually helps. In other parts, deliberately sparing the sore part pays. Remember that bursitis pain comes from rubbing raw surfaces together, and this rubbing itself makes the surfaces rawer still.

Leader guide inflammation. The commonest form of this complaint is excruciating soreness and swelling of the forearm when you have done a job which requires repeatedly making the same motion with your hand or wrist, like painting or driving nails. If you lay your other hand on the sore wrist, you may be able to feel a creaking like that of a leather saddle. Inflammation of the leaders' lubricated sheaths may strike in the hand or ankle, too. These miseries drag on and on unless you use intensive treatment, but they respond very well to these home measures:

Aspirin in the doses described above helps to keep you comfortable and to speed healing.

Splinting is absolutely necessary, and must extend to all of the parts which can be moved by the sore muscles. Tendon sheath inflammation in the wrist calls for bandaging the whole hand and wrist, for instance. I generally pad a light piece of board well and bind it to the top of the fingers, wrist and forearm with an elastic bandage.

Contrast baths three or four times a day are well worth the effort. See page 30 for specific directions.

CHAPTER THREE

How to Fight Diarrhea, Indigestion, Stomach Ulcers, and Gall Bladder Trouble

You seldom hear a North Country citizen complain of diarrhea or stomach upset, but the reason is a trick of language, not an iron-clad intestine. Any brief difficulty with the stomach or bowels is "stomach flu" to a Minnesotan. In spite of a phlegmatic temperament and uniformly clean kitchens, our Scandinavian and Deutschlander citizens have had lots of chance to try home remedies against indigestion and diarrhea. Instead of ignoring such discomfort until it goes away or taking some remedy you have seen advertised on TV, why don't you try the effective steps they have worked out over the years?

HOME REMEDIES FOR DIARRHEA

The outlander blames our smorgasbord, the native blames outlander's germs, but they both suffer the same miseries and need the same measures for relief when diarrhea strikes. Home treatment is often highly effective for loose or watery bowel movements, and is perfectly safe for any adult to try so long as there is no evidence of serious disease (such as pain which might be due to appendicitis).

The long fast. The most effective single method you can use to stop an attack of diarrhea is a period of absolute fasting. Whenever nausea or severe loss of appetite accompanies diarrhea, you will do better to omit even water the first six to twelve hours. If your stomach seems unaffected, you can take water, strained fruit juice, ginger ale, weak tea or clear broth. Moderately cooled beverages and lukewarm soup cause less cramps or upset than ice cold or hot liquids. You will find that very small quantities at frequent intervals sit better than a whole glassful or bowl at a time.

Bowel-flushing enemas. Strange as it seems, an enema often gives you a lot of relief and speeds your recovery from diarrhea. The germs that underlie most attacks actually die out very quickly, but the poisons they leave behind continue to irritate the bowel lining for some time. A thorough cleansing enema rids you of those poisons much more quickly and comfortably than more watery movements. One formula that usually does the job without stirring up hardly any cramping or discomfort is this:

Table salt	1 teaspoonful
Baking soda	2 teaspoonfuls
Warm water	1 quart

Use a small tip, well lubricated with petroleum jelly. Lie on your left side. Let the fluid run in slowly. Whenever you feel uncomfortably full or get any trace of a cramp, stop the flow, take several deep breaths and knead deeply but gently along the left side of your abdomen from below upward with the flat of your fingers. When the enema is complete, or when you find that further flow makes uncomfortable pressure even after a two minute rest with massage, you may expel it immediately. There is no need to hold in the solution to get full effect.

Most ordinary episodes of diarrhea respond to a single, thorough cleansing enema. In very severe attacks, two or three enemas at intervals of one to four hours may be needed. You can use cleansing enemas as often as recurrence of diarrhea and griping shows the need.

Fluid restoring enemas. The dragged-out feeling and fever which often accompany diarrhea stem partly from loss of body fluid. Watery stools can make diarrhea a serious illness even in adults, especially if nausea or vomiting keeps you from drinking anything. When an attack of diarrhea first starts, you should weigh yourself on an accurate scale. If the attack is severe, weigh yourself again at intervals through the day. If you lose more than five pounds or more than three per cent of your body weight, try taking one to four ounces of lukewarm water as an enema every 30 to 60 minutes. Deliver the fluid slowly. Press the cheeks of your buttocks together with both hands and lie still with your legs straight for five minutes or so afterward. Your body will soak the liquid up quickly. If your weight drops 5 to 8 pounds or 5 per cent, your doctor can probably speed your recovery with injections of fluid or with other prescription measures.

Diarrhea in children. Fluid loss causes special problems in infants and young children. Perhaps the easiest way to explain the problem is to look at a pound of our good Minnesota butter. Leave that pound in one piece and it has six surfaces—four sides, a top and a bottom. Cut it in half and the surface area is substantially increased—both cut surfaces are now added to the area already exposed.

The smaller the object the greater its surface per pound. This is true both of butter and human beings. There's an additional complication with children, though, because this principle applies to all kinds of surfaces, not just to the body's outside. A baby has many times more gut lining area per pound than an adult, and more lung lining, and more skin. Since he can lose fluid from all of these surfaces, fever and diarrhea dry him out in a hurry.

The best way to judge a child's or baby's water loss is by abrupt weight change, but if you don't have a sufficiently accurate scale you can use the *skin snap-back test*. You might check your youngsters with this technique right now, so you'll recognize any change from their normal. Just pinch up a fold of loose skin on an arm or abdomen and watch how quickly it springs back into place. If springback becomes definitely sluggish during an attack of diarrhea, best call your doctor—fluid injections may save a lot of difficulty later. For borderline sluggishness in snapback, try fluid replacement enemas of half an ounce to an ounce delivered with an infant syringe very slowly, and with the child's buttocks held together for five minutes afterward to make release less likely. A really dry youngster can soak up fluid from the rectum faster than you would believe— half an ounce to an ounce every half hour or so if necessary, and every hour in almost every case. I've seen many situations in which this much extra fluid kept a child from getting into the dehydration-fever-more-dehydration circle and prevented need for hospital-type injection care.

Don't neglect cleansing type enemas with youngsters, either. Use the same proportions of salt and soda with smaller quantities—two ounces for infants and four to eight ounces for older children—or use Fleet's Disposable Enema Kits (ready mixed, in a disposable plastic squeeze bottle) which come in both children's and adult sizes and cost less than a dollar at any drugstore.

Kaolin compounds. You can buy several preparations like Kaopectate or Pectocil which help to soak up poisons as they travel through the intestine. You will benefit from using a remedy of this type if your stomach is not too upset to permit it. However, the doses recommended on the bottle are almost always much too small. Pick a compound with no dangerous antispasmodics, the active ingredients being kaolin and pectin only, and take two tablespoonfuls at least four times a day for 24 to 48 hours.

Paregoric. You should not use paregoric for cramps which come every two or three minutes or if there is any one area of tenderness in your abdomen (particularly on the right) for fear of obscuring appendicitis. However, an adult can get quick relief from the griping pains that sometimes accompany diarrhea with one to two teaspoonfuls of paregoric repeated every six hours if necessary. Children six to twelve can take half a teaspoonful of paregoric, with dosages for younger children in the range of two drops for every ten pounds weight. Many patients get the same results with a bigger safety margin in dosage from Lomotil (R), available in any drug store without a prescription. Adults take two tablets four times a day until the situation is under control, and follow up with half doses for three days. Children do better with the liquid form, with dosage according to age. At 3-6 months the child needs 1/2 teaspoonful three times a day; 6 months to two years 1/2 teaspoonful four times a day; two to five years one teaspoonful three times a day; and 6 to 12 years one teaspoonful four times a day. Since paregoric or Lomotil slows movements of poison-laden material through your intestine, you should always use at least one cleansing enema inside a few hours after your first dose.

Stepwise reintroduction of foods. About half the patients who come to me for diarrhea have already virtually cured themselves once, then brought back the problem by eating solid food too quickly. You can help to speed and maintain your recovery from diarrhea by following this schedule:

Take nothing to eat or drink until at least two hours after onset of the diarrhea, or until four hours after any nausea or vomiting has ceased.

Start on moderately cooled or room temperature ginger ale, either straight or mixed with a little fruit juice. Sip this slowly from a small juice glass, taking at least ten minutes to down the first small serving. If this causes no upset, wait half an hour to an hour, then try another small portion. Continue small servings of ginger ale, fruit juice, weak tea or clear broth at quarter hour intervals until the diarrhea has been stopped for at least six hours, which will usually be about twelve hours from the onset of the illness.

At this point, take custards, soft boiled or poached eggs, toast, cooked cereal, and bland soups like chicken noodle or chicken rice.

Wait at least 24 hours before you eat ordinary food. If you get the least sign of nausea, diarrhea, or severe loss of appetite, quit food and liquid again for four to six hours and start back on liquids.

Salt. Watery stools wash a great deal of salt out of your system, with the result that you often feel weary and dragged out for days or weeks afterward. The best restorative for this post-diarrhea drag is plain table salt. Salt your foods heavily, put lots of salty meats and dishes on the menu. If you tire very, very easily, take heat-fatigue-type salt tablets three or four times a day for about a week.

Allergic diarrhea. If you have a food allergy, some ordinary foodstuffs which are completely harmless to other people may be digestive poisons to you. They almost always cause diarrhea, often with belching, gas pains, or vomiting. A tip-off to this condition is sometimes the undigested state of the food that passes: you may still be able to identify every item eaten. Another tip-off is that once the offending meal is gone the symptoms usually quit with no left-over weakness or loss of appetite. Most victims also have many relatives with hay fever, hives, asthma, or migraine.

Antihistamines. You may get at least partial relief from allergic diarrhea with the antihistamine formulas available without prescription. Your doctor may be willing to write a prescription for something stronger to keep in your medicine chest, too.

Paregoric.[1] Griping pain yields fairly well to paregoric in doses of one to two teaspoonfuls every four hours. If discomfort forces you to take paregoric, be sure to take an enema or a dose of salts two hours later to speed passage of the materials to which you are allergic.

Food and diarrhea records. You can entirely control episodes of allergic diarrhea in only one way: by finding out which foods cause your trouble and eliminating them from your diet. A written record of everything you have had to eat or drink within twenty-four hours before an attack is often very helpful, especially if you have only infrequent attacks. One of my patients used to get diarrhea and indigestion frequently during the Christmas and Easter seasons, but not at the rest of the year. When he kept written records, he easily traced his trouble to the citron in fruit cake and hot cross buns.

There is one danger in keeping a food diary: you may deprive

---

[1]A few states have made paregoric a prescription-only drug, because addicts sometimes distill the opium out of it. However, most doctors are willing to prescribe limited quantities for medicine chest use.

yourself of many foods which actually are harmless. If you find that you cannot avoid the foods to which you have seemed allergic without greatly limiting the variety of your diet, you should suspect hidden allergy to a common food like wheat, eggs or milk. Often you can eat a certain amount of such a food without developing complaints, so that you conclude that it is harmless. Then you get an attack from a large quantity of the food which is concealed as an ingredient in a pastry or food mixture, and blame the episode on some completely different substance. If your list gets too long, recheck by seeing whether each food on it will actually bring on an attack.

HOW TO CONTROL DIGESTIVE DISTRESS

You can relieve most mild or sporadic digestive distress for yourself, without a doctor's care. Before you try home measures, though, you should always ask yourself two questions:

1. Could this attack be appendicitis? Cramps from appendicitis often start in the pit of your stomach. Although they usually settle into your right side, pain and soreness often center on the left or up fairly high in the abdomen. If any one area of your abdomen is particularly tender in conjunction with abdominal cramps and either with or without nausea, appendicitis could be at fault. Certainly, you should check with your doctor within six hours after abdominal pain starts if you have not been able to obtain complete relief, even if the situation seems to be getting better. Be particularly alert for appendicitis in older children. Youngsters between nine and fourteen know enough about appendicitis to conceal symptoms from their parents in an effort to avoid an operation, but not enough to realize the danger of this course.

2. Have attacks been sufficiently regular to suggest a serious underlying cause? Indigestion which occurs two or three times a week for three weeks or more deserves medical attention even if it is easy to control with home measures. Such attacks sometimes stem from serious ulcers, tumor, or other illnesses for which your doctor can give considerably more aid if he sees you before the disease gets a head start.

If you can answer both these questions with a ringing "No," home remedies are worth a thorough trial. The proper approach varies according to whether your main complaint is heartburn, sick stomach, or gas and pressure pains.

Heartburn. A burning sensation or hot lump in the pit of the stomach fifteen to sixty minutes after a meal usually yields to *antacids* like baking soda, milk of magnesia or aluminum hydroxide. If you take baking soda, use one teaspoonful in half a glass of water. After about half an hour, if your symptoms are fairly well relieved, take a cup of warm milk or chocolate to keep down acid rebound. Milk of magnesia or aluminum hydroxide does not always give quite as good relief from the initial attack, but causes no acid rebound. They work very well for mild or early attacks. If you take aluminum hydroxide tablets, be sure to chew them thoroughly and take at least half a glass of water with each pill.

Sick stomach. If your main complaint is nausea, the key point is what you *eat and drink*. A thorough rest for your stomach through complete fasting generally helps. After about six hours, you can start on ginger ale or mixtures of ginger ale and fruit juice, not too cold, or on clear, lukewarm broth. If this sits well, you can start cooked cereal, soup, poached or boiled eggs, and toast after another six hours. Usually, it is wise to avoid ketchup, mustard and other strong seasonings for three to five days. Straight liquor or cocktails may stir up trouble, too, although tall drinks or wine usually do not.

Sleeping tablets. One of the best medicines for sick stomach is ordinary sleeping tablets. If you have some of these on hand, the dose recommended for bedtime use will usually quell your nausea at the price of only slight drowsiness if you stay on your feet. Take no more than half doses if you plan to operate a motor car or any hazardous machinery, though.

Prescription nausea fighters. Compazine and Thorazine work wonders with nausea and vomiting. You'll have to get your doctor on the phone to okay their use, since they are sold on prescription only. He'll tell you about dosage (which varies with your weight) and choose the right form (which varies with the length of action required).

If you have a lot of "24-hour stomach flu" around your area—brief attacks of vomiting without pain that sweep through the family—it's not a bad idea to get your doctor to okay a few Compazine suppositories for you to keep around the house. These allow you to follow the "complete rest for the system—nothing to eat or drink" rule and still get prompt medicinal relief. Just unwrap a suppository and insert it into the rectum blunt-end first. The medicine soaks in directly from your intestine, and usually controls nausea and vomiting within half an hour.

Gas and pressure pains. The best single measure here is a *carmina-*

tive enema. Be sure that no areas of tenderness or other signs of appendicitis or infection are present. Set up the enema bag and fill it with one quart of water at 115 degrees, which is about as hot as your fingers can stand. Add two teaspoonfuls of spirits of peppermint or tincture of asafetida. Allow the mixture to run in slowly, with pauses and deep breaths to allow griping or discomfort to subside. Try to retain this enema for three to five minutes, giving gentle kneading massage to the abdomen during this period.

In milder cases, or if there is any tenderness, a small *gas-moving enema* works better. This involves half a cup of warm water, a teaspoonful of glycerine, and a level tablespoonful of Epsom salts. Retain this enema for five to ten minutes if possible.

Suppositories. The highly effective spasm soothing ingredient of some hemorrhoidal suppositories makes them a good home substitute for prescription-only tablets and liquids. "Wyanoids" contain enough belladonna to soak in through the rectal lining and give relief throughout your entire intestinal tract. Insert one immediately after a carminative or gas-moving enema has been evacuated for extra prompt action.

Spasm soothers. Your doctor will probably be glad to have you keep some prescription type spasm soothers on hand in your medicine chest once he has picked a preparation and dosage which is one hundred per cent safe for you. If you have frequent difficulties, ask him what he recommends for your type of attack the next time you visit his office.

Low residue diet. If less material has to pass on through your intestine, cramp-causing spasms are less likely to develop. The main sources of indigestible fiber are raw vegetables, including most salad greens, the cabbage family (cabbage, brussels sprouts, and broccoli) and bran cereals. You often get considerable relief from cramps by omitting these foods.

Less milk. A few of my patients have complained of gassy indigestion for which all the usual measures gave little relief. On questioning, these people usually prove to subsist largely on dairy products—a quart or more of milk a day, plus considerable amounts of cheese and ice cream. By limiting their daily intake of dairy products to a pint of milk or its equivalent (two ounces of cheese or two servings of ice cream), many of these patients get complete relief. This much milk meets all your dietary needs as an adult, so you won't do yourself any harm to try it.

How to fight a tendency toward indigestion. If you are subject to indigestion, you can take many effective steps right in your own home to prevent attacks from getting a start. Both morale-boosting and physical measures definitely help. You should either make mealtimes cheerful times or adjust your meals to fit your mood and circumstances, besides using physical correctives.

Check family and business problems at the dining room door. Mealtime should be a time of relaxed enjoyment. You certainly help digestion when you make mealtime more mentally relaxed and more socially enjoyable.

The vice-president of a large publishing house met me once for luncheon. We had a pleasant meal, during which we discussed everything from Broadway plays to dry fly fishing. Then we went to his office for a business chat. As I was leaving, he said:

"A few years ago, I would have done this differently. Instead of just passing the time of day at luncheon and killing another half an hour getting our business settled, I would have gotten down to business with the main course. We would have signed a contract before dessert. Then I would have come up here and wrestled with indigestion for a solid hour!"

I've seen so many patients who followed that same futile routine! They do it with business affairs: if there's nobody to dicker with, they work away with reports and timetables when they should be enjoying a calm lunch. They do it with family affairs: they bicker all the way through a meal instead of setting a cooperative mood with the quiet companionship of the dinner table and then discussing their differences later. They even do it with completely private worries, fretting themselves into indigestion when a pleasant mealtime interlude might help them try to find a fresh, productive approach. Wouldn't it be much better to do as my publisher friend now does? To use mealtime for pleasant personal exchange and relaxed enjoyment, then make a fresh attack upon your problems?

Build pleasant conversation. Properly guided conversation inevitably sets a good, digestion-aiding mood at mealtime. The trick is to lead your companions gently toward topics that interest or stimulate them. One of the best conversationalists I know blames his success on the morning newspaper, a red pencil, and a ten-minute wait between buses every day. He scans the paper quickly, learning just enough about each headline to know what it is about and whom it might interest.

"I don't know the answers," he says. "All I know is the right questions to ask or the right issues to raise."

That's all it takes to avoid dull silence, arguments, or embarrassment during mealtimes. You can get your husband talking with a remark like, "Which do you think is the team to watch in pro football this year?" You can steer conversation away from a topic that might lead to hard feelings by referring to a new subject which interests the other person: the latest dress styles, or the effect of union racketeering on labor. Such a stock of fresh topics with which to draw out your companions takes only a few minutes a day to accumulate.

Make meals more alluring. You can help your stomach to make more of its precious digestive juice by making meals and mealtime more alluring. Actual measurements prove that the flow of gastric juices increases dramatically when you look at an appetizing meal. More gastric juices pour into your stomach when you *look* at attractively prepared food than when you actually *taste* it. This extra flow of gastric juice becomes more and more important as the years go by and stomach juices become scanty. Yet many people take less and less trouble with sprucing up their meals as they grow older.

Margaret Bradshaw was a good example. Her husband died when she was fifty. For the next four years, she was plagued by indigestion. Yet she was cheerful, had many friends and few worries.

Margaret Bradshaw was too busy making a new life to spend time fixing attractive meals for herself. When she took work as housekeeper-companion for an elderly relative, she conscientiously dressed up the meals she served for her employer and herself. Result: an almost instant end to indigestion.

Fit meals to your mood. When you are in the grip of any strong emotion, such as anger, fear or excitement, or if the circumstances in which you eat may lead to such feelings, you should not eat heavy or hard-to-digest foods. You can either delay meals or simplify and lighten them. One of my patients, for instance, had a violent temper and an acrimonious wife. For years, not only his household but also his abdomen were in perpetual uproar. But no longer. He has finally learned to skip meals when he is angry. He storms out of the house at least once a week, walks the streets until he calms down, then takes a bowl of cream-style soup every hour or two until his stomach stops churning. Without the miseries of indigestion, he is making real progress toward a more pleasant life.

Better teeth for good digestion. Frequent, severe attacks of indigestion often stem from poor teeth or inadequate chewing. Take Hilda Swanson's case, for example. At age sixty-three, Hilda was spending nearly a hundred dollars a year at the drug store. Her life was a never-ending succession of poached eggs, milk toast, and misery. Heartburn and gas pains plagued her when she tried to eat solid foods, constipation tortured her when she didn't. Yet there was nothing wrong with Hilda's stomach or bowel. Half a dozen examinations and several X-rays had been entirely normal.

Poor Hilda! She spent so much on pills and potions that she had nothing left for her teeth. Her smile was a jagged horror. Only two pairs of teeth in her head met in any kind of bite. Her appearance finally drove her children into arranging for her dentist to fit her with plates. To everyone's surprise, her digestion improved overnight once she had effective teeth. Today, Hilda enjoys her food again. She hardly ever takes a pill, and thanks God that her children were worried about her jagged smile.

Food to fit your teeth. Suit your food choices to your teeth. If your teeth can't be fixed so that you can chew everything easily, you'll have to give in to them. Follow these simple rules:

1. Take hard-to-bite foods in a different form. Instead of eating a whole apple, have it cut up in salad or fruit cup.

2. Morsel food before eating it. If you get a tough piece of meat, cut a thin piece against the grain, then slice across it several times with the grain before gathering a bite with your fork.

Soften food in preparation. Get the butcher to tenderize meat and grind your hamburger twice. Have steaks thoroughly pounded before they are cooked. Be sure that vegetables are slightly overcooked to soften their fiber.

Take time to chew. Give yourself time to eat calmly, time to chew well, and time to enjoy your meals. I've seen many a case of indigestion cured by the simple advice to chew each bite at least ten times. The first week a patient follows this rule, he concentrates on counting. After that, he discovers flavor, leisurely enjoyment of food, new satisfaction at the table and misery-free digestion. He doesn't have to count any more. He chews automatically.

Low acidity indigestion. If you have stomach bloating, fullness, belching, and discomfort after meals, you may suffer from lack of stomach acid. Properly diluted hydrochloric acid just before and during meals often gives tremendous relief. Buy *dilute* hydrochloric acid, also called 0.1 N, at your drugstore, put ten drops in a glass of water and set it on the table with each meal. Sip the solution through a glass straw with its tip well inside your teeth on top of your tongue to avoid possible dental damage. Take a sip or two before beginning to eat, and repeat at intervals throughout the meal.

Caffeine spurred indigestion. As few as three cups of coffee a day or equivalent amounts of tea or cola beverages can cause digestive disturbances over a period of time in sensitive people. Digestive effects are slow to appear and slow to leave: it takes three weeks of overindulgence to cause trouble, and almost as long to improve after you cut down on coffee-drinking. Patients who get well after a switch to decaffeinated coffee often had no indigestion until after age forty, even though they had been drinking lots of coffee since age twenty or so. They almost never complain of coffee nerves.

If there's any chance that caffeine might be troubling your digestion, switch to decaffeinated coffee for a month. You can continue to drink regular coffee in restaurants or in other people's homes so long as you keep it down to one or two cups a day. At the end of the first month, the harmful caffeine effects should be about gone. See whether the next week or two are brightened by better digestion. If they are, keep dodging excess caffeine for life.

Worms. When I first started in practice, I remember puzzling over one of the Olson brood. Young Sam had stomach aches and side aches two or three times a week. He cidn't eat hearty the way a twelve-year-old should. But his blood count and x-rays were perfectly all right, and I couldn't seem to find a cure.

One day the boy's grandmother was confined to bed, so I went out to see her. The house was spic and span, without a speck of dirt, and Grandma was propped between snowy sheets. I checked her out and prescribed for her. As I got ready to leave, her daughter asked me to take a look at Sam, who was having "another of his attacks." I looked the boy over and suggested another crop of x-rays.

"X-rays?" Grandmother snorted from her sickbed. "Why in my day we'd have cured that boy six months ago. Give him a good slug of worm medicine and that would be the end of it."

You know what? She was one hundred per cent right! Knowing how scrubbed and spic and span the Olson house was, it never occurred to me that young Sam might have worms. But I know better now, and the first thing I do when a youngster complains of stomach pains or loss of appetite is check a bit of stool under the microscope to see if it contains worm eggs. It happens in the best of families, and without anyone making any breech in cleanliness or proper care!

Prescription measures work so much better than home remedies on the various types of worms that I'm not going to advise how you can treat them. But doctors are squeamish about checking for this condition, especially when they know you run a clean household and might be offended by the suggestion. You often have to take the initiative in getting the proper studies done. Particularly if your youngster has suggestive complaints or if you live in a warm, moist climate, catch a bit of stool and take it in when any of your youngsters sees a doctor. You'll be surprized at how often stubborn, smoldering difficulties stem from easily cured infestation with worms.

HOME CARE FOR ULCERS AND GASTRITIS·

If you get heartburn or boring pain in the pit of your stomach at least once a day an hour or two after meals, you probably have either gastritis or an ulcer. Any digestive complaints which last more than three weeks deserve a medical checkup, of course. However, prompt home care may get the problem under control before expensive X-rays and doctor visits become worthwhile. Exactly the same home care often cures either gastritis or beginning ulcer, so you can use these remedies whenever you have suggestive complaints:

Simplified ulcer-healing diet. You can usually bring an ulcer or attack of gastritis under control promptly by taking six small meals of very bland foods a day. Eat cooked cereal, soft boiled or poached eggs, toast, butter, strained cream soups, custards, puddings, or plain cookies. You can eat ice cream, too, it you let it melt in your mouth before you swallow it.

Acid-absorbing milk. While you are healing your ulcer or gastritis, you need something to neutralize stomach acids as quickly as they form. Milk is the best answer. Half a glass of whole milk or of half-milk-half-cream every hour except at mealtime does the trick. For a change-off and at bedtime, try flavored Swiss or French style yogurt. This has the same acid-neutralizing and nutritional qualities as milk, in a variety of flavors. The more solid consistency helps to keep it in your stomach a little longer, which is especially helpful for neutralizing night acids.

Antacids. If the six-feeding diet and the milk portions between do not keep you entirely comfortable, try aluminum hydroxide tablets between milk feedings. These tablets are available without prescription under various brand names such as "Gelusil" and "Amphogel." Chew well and take them with water. As your condition improves, you still need something to neutralize stomach acids every 90 minutes during the day for several weeks. Aluminum hydroxide often proves much more convenient than milk. Try it at first alternating with milk, then as your acid-fighting mainstay.

Milk of magnesia. With little solid food and lots of constipating milk and medicine, most gastritis victims find that their bowels get rather tight. Since milk of magnesia acts both as an antacid and as a mild laxative, you can usually keep your bowels going by replacing one or two doses of aluminum hydroxide with milk of magnesia each day. Don't strive for daily movements, though. As long as the material is easily passed and is formed in normal sausage shapes, even one movement a week is sufficient.

Convalescent diet. After you have freed yourself of digestive discomfort for a week, you can usually go back to a three meal program. You should probably stay off of seasonings, spices, and alcohol for good. Let hot foods cool somewhat before eating them, and let cold foods warm in your mouth before you swallow. Choose stewed or roasted meat over broiled whenever possible, and avoid fried foods altogether. Try to get your vegetables cooked a bit longer than usual so that they will be soft, and chew them thoroughly. Keep taking at least one glassful of milk between meals and in the evening for several months or years.

How to keep an ulcer from coming back on you. If you have a tendency toward ulcer or gastritis, you can usually take effective measures to keep further attacks from plaguing you.

Precautions under stress. When you know that you are under extra emotional stress or when you get into an upsetting situation, you can often ward off an ulcer attack by anticipating it. In mildly distressing situations, simply eating half a cup of yogurt at bedtime each night may do the trick. Night acids are the first to increase when an ulcer threatens, and yogurt sticks in the stomach long enough to neutralize at least the worst of these. In times of greater stress, go on your full six meal program with milk or antacid every hour for two or three days. That's easier than letting the ulcer get a fresh start.

Build an ulcer-dodging way of life. Even the worst ulcers can be prevented by a happy choice of attitude. That's what an Iowa internist proved a few years ago when he got tired of treating the same patients over and over again for ulcers. He picked the very worst cases, people who had suffered at least three recent bouts with ulcer. Then he asked each of them something like this:

"Want to spend one night a month trying to keep from getting another attack? No pills, no shots, no treatments: just come in for a quiet chat with some other people who have the same sort of problems. Together, maybe you can work out a better way to reduce or meet the stresses of life."

Over thirty patients took him up on it. They met after normal office hours and talked about effectual, contented living. Seven years later, my friend counted up the score. Without the conferences, these patients should have suffered at least forty ulcer bouts, many of them severe. With the conferences, only four mild attacks had developed.

You can promote ulcer-dodging, digestion-improving attitudes in yourself. Only extreme cases, like the ulcer-ridden unfortunates my Iowa friend assembled, need expert help in working out a new viewpoint. You can probably decide for yourself whether your attitudes need any changes, and if so act accordingly.

Decide how much to depend on others emotionally and how much to let them depend on you. The main key to freedom from digestion-wrecking stress is just the right balance between self-reliance on the one hand, and genuine concern for others and need for their loving support on the other. You need to feel that others depend on you. You also need to depend on *them*—to yearn for and receive evidence of their concern.

You can easily develop such two-way support and need without losing control of your own destiny or confidence in your own powers. The secret is compassion: emotional sharing of each other's trials. Advice and even actual aid are sometimes threats: they can hamper self-reliance and destroy self-confidence. Compassion is no threat. You can feel for others and let them know that you are behind them without taking over their decisions or putting them in your debt. You can share and discuss feelings which upset you without asking advice or aid.

How Bill Harper built himself a web of ulcer-healing emotional bonds. Bill Harper wore all the trappings of success when he first visited my office: a tailored suit, a diamond ring, and the miserable, drawn expression of perennial ulcer suffering.

"I've always been a battler," he told me toward the end of his visit. "I've fought for business, fought for social position, fought for community standing. Why should that give ·me an ulcer, though? I usually win!"

"Fighting for things doesn't cause ulcers," I told him. "It's the insecurity that makes you *have* to fight. What makes you a battler? Why can't you enjoy the fruits of each success instead of moving on?"

"I can't answer that. I'm just that kind of a guy."

"Don't you think some of your drive comes from dissatisfaction? How about your family life, for instance?"

"I'm proud of my family—I'd do anything for them, and they'd do anything for me."

"Is that enough?"

Bill Harper looked at me thoughtfully. "I'll think about that," he said, and left.

The next time we talked about family life was nearly a year afterward.

"My wife made me very happy today," Bill said.

"How?" I asked.

"She told me what has been troubling her recently. She's worried sick about our girl going steady already at age seventeen."

He smiled ruefully, then went on:

"A year ago she wouldn't have come to me. And if she had, I wouldn't have known what to do, except send them both on a trip to Bermuda or something. We've come a long way since then: she told me because she knew I'd be concerned, and I guess we both felt better afterward."

Bill Harper hasn't had any more trouble with his ulcer. He's found new, lasting satisfaction in his home, with truly deep emotional attachments to replace the selfish, pragmatic pride of yesteryear. The same change improves his friendships and even his business contacts. Without in any way decreasing his success, he's put his life on a sounder emotional footing, and enjoyed both psychological and physical benefits.

Learn to say, "No." Next to proper balance of self-reliance and close, mutual concern, the most important key to freedom from digestion-wrecking stress is ability to say "no." It's altogether too easy to drift into a harried, over-burdened ineffectiveness by saying "yes" to whatever anyone asks you to do.

A distinguished community leader and old family friend made this point for me in an unexpected way. When I was in my twenties, he asked me to take on a responsibility I didn't want. I hated to refuse such an old and respected friend, so I hedged. After several miserable days of stalling, I finally said "no."

"Thank Heaven!" my friend replied. "You've finally arrived!"

"What do you mean?" I asked.

"You've taken your place as a man. Until the day you first say 'no' to someone or something you like, you're just a piece of human jetsam, floating with the tides of man's demands. Now you're setting your own course. Congratulations!"

That moment comes back to me whenever I see an overburdened sufferer from abdominal distress. To get him well more quickly, I usually tell him to stop all of his activities and responsibilities except one or two. Then as he starts to pick up the threads again, I say:

"Pick and choose. Of course you want to help everybody who

asks, but you can't. So figure all the responsibilities you have—family, business, household, and community—before you take on a new job or join another group. Can you add this without taking away from something else? If not, what do you want to drop to make room for it?

"Ask yourself these questions, and you'll find yourself saying 'no' to many offers. But don't feel badly about it. You're giving yourself more thoroughly, as well as enjoying yourself much more, if you stick to the jobs which really fit you as a person, and fit your stores of energy and time."

Most harried, dyspeptic people find this advice worthwhile. Does it suit your situation?

Evade or rid yourself of resentment. You can frequently ease some digestion-wrecking stress by evading or releasing resentment. Several years ago, Drs. Wolf and Wolfe studied digestion in a patient who had an opening directly into his stomach. The man was hired as a janitor at the hospital, partly so that he would be available for the doctors' experiments. He wasn't a very good janitor: he was often called on the carpet. But that seemed to make very little difference to his stomach.

Then one day, it did make a difference. The inside of his stomach was beet-red in places, blotchy, sensitive and raw.

"What's happened to you, Tom?" the doctors asked.

"Just a bawling out," the patient said. But further questioning revealed one special point: this bawling out was for something not his fault. This bawling out he deeply resented, knowing it was undeserved, while he had taken others as a matter of course.

Is your stomach ever upset, sensitive, and uncomfortable? If so, seek back for sources of resentment. You'll find that you will want to dodge some similar stresses in the future as simply not worth the upsetting effect they have on you. Other resentments fade when you talk them over with your family or friends. Still others rankle until you develop some safety-valve activity—a hobby or sports interest that lets you cut or chop, hit a ball, or shoot down a bird. Emotion ceases to cause ulcers when it has an easy outlet, even though that outlet is through conversation or assault on wood or leather. For complete details, see pages 217-218.

BILIOUS INDIGESTION, AND GALL BLADDER DISEASE AND STONE

Bilious indigestion responds very well to simple home measures, as long as you do not have true gall-bladder colic. Colic shows up as cramp-like pain below the edge of your right ribs. The cramps come about every two minutes and last ten seconds or so (although it seems much longer). They may run through to your back, right under your shoulder blade. Nausea or vomiting often adds its miseries to the colicky pain. Since gallstones frequently underlie attacks of colic, prompt prescription measures are definitely worthwhile once cramps occur. Otherwise, home treatment may bring your problem promptly under control.

Are you subject to gall bladder trouble? One good thing about gall bladder trouble: the people who are most subject to it can find out about their predisposition in advance and take extra precautions. Determine your gall bladder index as follows:

First, look at the boundary between your chest and your abdomen. If the edge of the chest bones forms a very sharp angle, you are unlikely to have gall bladder trouble. If your lower ribs form a very blunt angle, gall bladder trouble is quite likely to plague you. Find the angle closest to your own in Figure One, and score the corresponding number toward your gall baldder index.

Second, check your coloring. Blonde, fair-skinned people are much more prone to suffer gall bladder trouble than brunettes. Score six points if you are very fair, four points if you are blondish or redheaded and two points if you are fair-complexioned regardless of hair color.

Third, take your sex into account. Women are several times as likely to get gall bladder trouble as men, and should add four points to their gall bladder index.

If your gall bladder index totals ten or more, you should take extra precautions against gall bladder disease. What kind of precautions?

1. Drink enough water to ward off thirst. Studies prove that gall bladder sufferers seldom put water on the table and drink much less fluid than other people. There's no need to flood your system beyond nature's expressed needs, but you should serve water with each meal and heed any slight twinge of thirst at or between mealtimes.

2. Eat at mealtime only. Your gall bladder holds your body's reserve supply of bile, which should pile up only from one meal to another. When you divide your body's daily fuel into three nearly equal portions, each of them is large enough to make your gall bladder empty itself. When you scatter your food intake by tasting during food preparation, by picking between meals, or by taking a succession of snacks, thick bile stagnates. Irritation of the gall bladder results. Gallstones are more likely to form.

3. Try to enjoy foods through better seasoning instead of extra richness. If your build, coloring, and sex make you especially subject to gall bladder trouble, you are almost immune to ulcers or stomach irritation. You can use spices and savory sauces quite safely. Rich foods, on the other hand, have

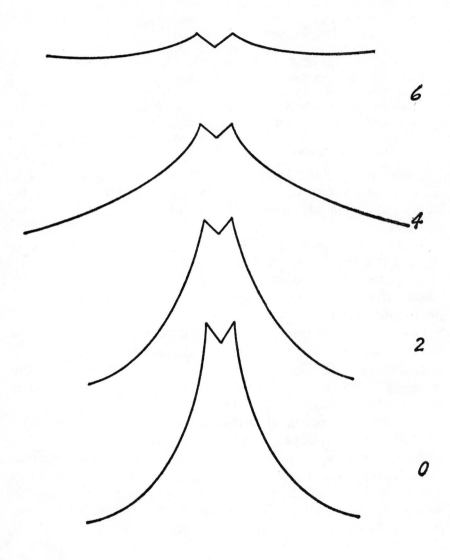

Figure One: *Add in the number beside the rib angle closest to your own in calculating your gall bladder index. Split the difference if you can't tell which of two angles is closest.*

extra risks for potential gall bladder sufferers. Gallstones, with which one woman in four is afflicted by age forty, are formed from the cholesterol which your body makes from fat, most of which you eat in the form of fried foods and pastries.

4. Walk at least two miles a day, or take an equivalent amount of other, similar exercise. Lazy gall bladder type indigestion, often followed by stone formation, occurs mainly in people who remain physically inactive.

5. Spices, onions, and savory sauces add lingering odors and tastes to stomach gases. Bilious indigestion or gall bladder trouble causes belching at times, and when this occurs the sufferer usually tastes the spices, onions, and so on from his last meal. He falsely blames these "repeaters" for his trouble. If you are subject to belching attacks and find the flavoring of "repeaters" is itself unpleasant, cut them out. These substances are not really at fault, however; continuing to enjoy them will not usually make you belch more or cause further digestive troubles.

Bilious indigestion. When you get gas cramps, bloating, and belching after eating fried food or pork, your difficulty may be bilious indigestion. Many patients get considerable relief from home measures.

Enemas and suppositories. A carminative enema (one quart of water at 115 degrees with two teaspoonfuls of spirits of peppermint), followed by a Wyanoid suppository gives prompt relief from most bilious attacks (For further details see p. 52.) Prescription type spasm soothers may give benefit, too.

Low fat diet. A low fat diet helps ward off further attacks of bilious indigestion. Fried foods, pork, rich pastries, and oil-containing dressings must go. Replace cream with half and half, avoid whipping cream and keep butter down to one or two pats a day. Eat plenty of lean broiled or boiled meat, vegetables, and fruit.

Bile salts. Some patients find that they get considerable relief from bile salts (Bilron, Anabile, or any of several other brands). One tablet with each meal usually helps to keep the bowels active and prevents some bloating and gas pain. These tablets cause no heartburn or bitter belching if you take them during the meal rather than on an empty stomach, and swallow them whole. *But* remember that so-called liver pills are *not* adequate sources of bile salts, and are not recommended.

Laxative salts. You get better bile flow as well as relief from constipation with a dose of Phospho-soda or Epsom salts. Although these agents should not usually be used for ordinary constipation (see Chapter Four), they work very effectively for the constipation that accompanies biliousness. In fact, the effect on bile flow probably makes a dose worth-while whenever you miss your movement for 48 hours, if bilious indigestion is continually with you.

Serious gall bladder trouble. If you get proper medical care at the first sign of gall bladder colic, you may actually escape the need for surgery. As long as gallstones are very small or the gall bladder is only inflamed instead of packed with stones, your doctor may be able to prescribe diet and medicines that will help.

How to make a gall bladder operation easier to bear. If other methods fail or if your case is not suited to them, an operation almost always cures gall bladder trouble. You can make this operation much safer and easier to bear in three ways:

1. Get medical treatment from the start. Some people suffer through one attack of gallstone colic after another without a doctor's help because they are afraid that as soon as they call a doctor, he will operate. A doctor's help during and after early attacks may ward off the need for surgery. If it doesn't do that, it will keep you in good condition to undergo operation with less risks and difficulties.

2. Lose any excess weight. As soon as you have any suspicion that your gall bladder may be causing trouble, get your doctor to help you with a weight reduction plan. If you are overweight, the risks and miseries of surgery can be cut in half simply by getting to normal weight beforehand.

3. Go ahead with the operation before complications arise. Gallstones can work into the main bile passages, causing jaundice and other severe problems. I've never seen a patient who had severe complications without several preceding gallstone colics. If you heed your body's painful warnings and your doctor's sound advice, you can avoid these extra miseries, risks and disabilities.

How Mrs. Simpson made her operation easier to bear. Olive Simpson was crying when I first saw her.

"It's not the pain," she said as she dabbed at her eyes with the corner of the pillow case. "I'm just scared. My sister had her gall bladder out, and she had such an awful time!"

Olive had gall bladder colic which was due to large-sized stones. She needed an operation to get a cure, but her first attack settled down promptly. She had plenty of time to lose weight and get ready for surgery. When Olive went to the hospital four months later, she had lost forty pounds. She was as strong and healthy as she had ever been (her sister had waited until she was weak with jaundice).

"No operation is a picnic," Olive told me afterwards. "But when I think of what my sister went through, I'm mighty grateful for the easy time I had. There was just one day when I needed shots to ease my pain after surgery, and I got back on my feet in a tenth of the time it took her."

CHAPTER FOUR

How to Prevail Over Constipation

If constipation has never plagued you you have been fortunate indeed. Most people need to give definite attention to their bowel function at fairly frequent intervals, if not continually. Yet you can almost always control constipation completely with home measures. By steering clear of the easy but temporary means of relief, you can correct constipation without irritating your bowel and perpetuating your difficulty. Throw your convenient but ultimately harmful laxative pills out the window and try this effective, step-by-step program for total correction of a tight bowel.

STEP-BY-STEP CORRECTION OF TIGHT BOWELS

Step One: Give your bowel a rest on a low-bulk diet. Your bowel has probably been irritated by laxatives, overworked by bulk-formers, or scraped insensitive by dry bulk passages. Let it rest and heal itself for about two weeks before trying to achieve unaided, comfortably regular movements. A low-bulk diet provides the rest phase of your constipation cure. You can eat freely of meat, dairy products, eggs, and bread. Eat two normal servings of fruit or juice a day, one of lemon, orange, or grapefruit and one of bananas, pears, peaches, peeled apricots, baked apple, or strawberries. Also eat two servings of well-cooked peas, string beans, carrots, beets, spinach, tomato or potato.

During this time, you should take a *salt and soda enema* whenever you have discomforts like headache, nausea and cramps, or whenever you go more than three days without a movement. Follow this technique for a comfortable effective enema:

Dissolve one teaspoonful of table salt and two teaspoonfuls of baking soda in one quart of lukewarm water. Place in an enema bag. Use the smallest enema tip. Lubricate well with petroleum jelly. Lie on your left side, and insert the tip just far enough that it stays. Gradually raise the enema bag until it is one to two feet above the level of the enema tip, and let the mixture flow in gently. If abdominal discomfort develops, lower the bag somewhat and gently knead the left lower portion of your abdomen with your free hand. When the enema has all run in, remove the tip and prepare for an evacuation. As soon as an urge develops, the enema is working fully: you need not try to hold back.

Some patients find that somewhat larger enemas are perfectly comfortable and extra effective. If you feel that evacuations produced by one quart enemas are not adequate, put double quantities in the enema bag and run in as much as you can comfortably absorb.

On the other hand, if full-sized enemas cause too much discomfort or if your circumstances (such as often being away from home overnight) make them inconvenient, a Fleet's Disposable Enema Kit or a similar product is available without a prescription in any drugstore at modest cost. A special concentration of salt substances makes a few ounces of solution do a good job for most victims of constipation, and the outfit (with a plastic squeeze bottle and ready-lubricated tip) is completely ready to use.

If movements have been hard and massive, you can ease their passage with *preliminary internal oiling*. Place two ounces of warm olive oil into the rectum with a rubber ear or infant syringe half an hour or more before preparing the salt and soda solution or using Fleet's Kit.

Step Two: Gradually increase moist-bulk foods. When you have achieved a rested, irritation-free bowel, your next step is to increase gradually the amount of *moist-bulk producing* fruit you eat each day. Milder, never-irritating fruits should be chosen first. These are stewed prunes, cantaloupe or honeydew melon, raisins, currants, applesauce, plums, cherries, and berries.More irritating fruits like figs and dates are often very helpful, but must be tried at first with caution. If you have a sensitive bowel, they may do more harm than good. Raw apples must also be used with caution: they often cause gas in the presence of sluggish bile flow or gall bladder trouble.

During the moist-bulk increasing phase, most sufferers find that they need a little *mild lubricating or moisturizing medicine* for their bowel. A tablespoonful twice a day of any mineral oil emulsion like Petrolagar or Petromul does the trick. Be sure you use the plain emulsion, without added phenolphthalein or cascara. Moisture-holding colloids like Mucilose or Metamucil also do an excellent job. Take one heaping teaspoonful in a glass of water morning and

evening at first, following each dose with a full glass of water. A
higher or lower dose may work better for you, but wait several days
before deciding what you need. Meanwhile, use enemas if you get
very uncomfortable. The dose can be cut down gradually over a
period of weeks as natural moist-bulk foods take over your body's
requirements.

If abdominal comfort and easily-passed stools cannot be achieved
by these means, you probably need *spasm-relaxing medicines* or
other special measures. Wyanoids suppositories will give some benefit, until you can get your doctor to prescribe tablets or liquids. But
remember that your aim is comfort, not stools of a certain size or
frequency. Most people who fail at this point get discouraged
because they have small, infrequent stools—a natural effect of
low-bulk eating. Forget false notions about needing a bowel movement every day or every two days The key to a better-working
bowel is regulation that fits in with *your* body's natural patterns
without nausea, headache, bloating, cramps, or difficult-to-pass, hard
stools. Even if your natural rhythm proves to produce only one
movement a week, you should be content so long as that movement
is normally sausage-shaped and you do not suffer gas pains
beforehand.

**Step Three: Free yourself gradually of all bowel-regulating medi-
cines.** Medicines are only a crutch to keep you comfortable until new
mental, physical, and food habits solve your bowel problem. However, any abrupt change may throw your bowel out of kilter.
Medicines should be tapered slowly, taking a dose every single day,
but decreasing the dose very gradually over a period of six to eight
weeks. You may need an occasional enema during this time if you
cut down your medicine too quickly. Don't be discouraged. If you
taper slowly enough, you will almost always ultimately get along
without any medicines at all, and with very infrequent enemas.

*How Mrs. Harris followed the three steps to natural rhythm
regulation.* Mrs. Harris had taken laxatives every two or three days
for more than twenty years.

"Lots of doctors have told me to quit laxatives," she told me.
"But if I don't take something, I get miserable. Headache, gas pains,
upset stomach—it's more than I can bear."

Mrs. Harris followed the three step program we've just discussed.
When she set her bowel at rest with a low bulk diet and enemas, she
remained entirely comfortable. During Step Two she took a full
tablespoonful of Metamucil twice a day at first, and tapered very

slowly. She got used to eating fruit with each meal. At the end of four months, she was freed forever of the need for laxatives, and settled into a regular, comfortable bowel rhythm with two or three movements a week.

CONSTIPATION IN CHILDREN

When a mother brings a child into my office witn the complaint of constipation, the first thing I want to know is whether the *child* complained or whether the nature and frequency of movements upset the *mother.* Infrequent movements alone don't upset *me.* Stomach aches or loss of appetite (with or without constipation) make me want to check a stool specimen for worm eggs before I treat bowel rhythm. After sorting out these separate problems, though, I still find quite a few youngsters with constipation.

The toughest job we adults have with these youngsters is convincing them that cola drinks and candy don't "make it." Colas contain just as much caffeine as coffee, and have two harmful effects. Caffeine often throws the bowel into spasm and causes constipation. It always increases the flow of fluid through your kidneys and dries out your system instead of supplying needed internal moisture. Candy creates problems in a different way—not for what it is, but for what it replaces. Every candy bar kills the appetite as thoroughly as two or three pieces of fruit, for instance, and provides neither bulk nor moisture. It's hard to make these points without sounding like an old fogy, but maybe you can accomplish at least something by making your household purchases according to these rules. If youngsters can get ginger ale and fresh fruit out of the refrigerator for nothing, maybe they'll spend a little less of their "own money" on the less desirable alternatives.

Parents often have difficulty getting themselves to give their children an enema. It may be easier to spread some newspaper or other padding on the bathroom floor to administer the solution than it is to transport the child from the bedroom after giving the solution. Youngsters below age twelve do well with a pint of salt and soda solution (half quantities of each ingredient) or with a child's size Fleet's Enema. The former has the advantage that it can be expelled immediately, while the disposable kit solution has to be retained 5 minutes. In smaller children, glycerine suppositories (obtainable without a prescription) often give temporary relief just as effectively as an enema with a lot less bother. Keep these in the refrigerator or else they get too soft to insert readily. Unwrap and insert blunt-end first, then get the child to hold the suppository in for five minutes or so.

Infants need formula change for constipation, so you should call your doctor.

HOW TO FIGHT THE NATURAL TENDENCY TOWARD CONSTIPATION

Even if constipation has never plagued you enough to require a full-scale program for correction, you will probably find that measures to avoid it are worthwhile at times. Several techniques are easy to work into your daily way of life without consuming extra time, effort or money:

How to empty your lower bowel efficiently. You may make bowel movements much easier by following these simple toileting rules:

Take plenty of time, at the same time every day. After breakfast, or whenever you find movements most frequent, set aside 10 or 15 minutes for elimination. At first you may rarely have movements at this time. But if you persist your body will train itself to take advantage of the opportunity.

Read, listen to a portable radio, or relax mentally during toileting. Worry and tension clamp down your bowel into a stiff, inactive tube. Keep yourself distracted from concerns of the past or future while you're encouraging nature's call.

Flexed hips help your belly muscles work better at the toilet; a 6" or 8" footstool under your feet often makes elimination much easier.

Exercise. Your abdominal muscles, contracting in the course of everyday activity, massage the bowel. This massage helps to move bowel contents along until they can be eliminated. If you walk 10 to 20 blocks each day, the resulting muscular action makes your bowels move more freely.

Abdominal massage. If you do not have time to exercise, you can easily use your hands to replace muscular massage as follows:

Lie down and let your abdominal muscles go entirely loose. Place your right hand on the lowest part of the abdomen to the right of center. Press the little finger side firmly down into the abdomen. Roll your hand slowly toward the thumb side, as if you were kneading margarine along inside a sack. Place your left hand adjoining. Press the little finger side in, then roll toward the thumb side. Massage in this fashion up the right side of the abdomen, across the upper part, and down the left side. Then begin again low on the right. Continue massage for about five minutes.

Dodge dry bulk. Moist-bulk foods have always been the constipation victim's first standby. Fruits and cooked vegetables add moisture-holding bulk, and extra moisture makes movements easier. But it's the moisture that does the trick, not the bulk. Extra bulk in any form means extra work for your bowel, and dry bulk means extra work without extra moisture or other benefit.

Any victim of constipation should avoid these dry-bulk forming foods like the plague:

> Raw vegetables, especially rabbit-food type salads.
> Cabbage, brussels sprouts, and broccoli.
> Bran cereals.

Less tension means less constipation. Another effective way to fend off constipation is to relieve the tension which so often brings it on.

"When my wife helps me pack," one traveling man told me, "she'll stand there with my bottle of laxative pills and say: 'Is this trip going to be a chore or a pleasure?' If I say chore, she throws them in. If it's pleasure I never have the need."

If you control or air tensions you'll have much less trouble with constipation. You *can* control tension, usually without the aid of drugs or medicines. Simple home measures can help greatly in bringing tranquil calmness to your daily life.

How to hold up better under tension. You'll find that one controllable human trait adds greatly to tension: trying to grapple with the past or future in some corner of your mind at the same time that you attack the problems or manage the tasks of the present moment. While you cook the supper, you try to figure what you should have said in yesterday's argument, or you try to plan tomorrow's meals. While you do your job, you try to figure out how you got so far behind on your bills or what to get your wife for Christmas. The human mind is not meant to grapple with the separate problems of the past, the present, and the future at one time.

You can worry less and accomplish more if you take up problems one at a time. Live right now. Occupy your mind by chatting with your husband, listening to the radio, or adding other pleasant stimulations to the present moment. Then take time out: forget about right now and plan for later. Grapple with the present and the future separately instead of both at once, and forget most problems from the past.

TEMPORARY RELIEF WITHOUT LONG-RANGE HARM

If your bowel gets tight, you need relief. Most ordinary laxatives lead you into a vicious circle, though. They give temporary relief, but they irritate the lining of your bowel sufficiently that further tightness often develops. You can often keep yourself from getting into a really prolonged bout with constipation simply by sticking to these measures for temporary relief:

Enemas. A salt and soda enema, given according to the directions above, will never cause further bowel irritation or self-perpetuating constipation. Use enemas as often as necessary for relief of occasional costive spells.

Disposable enema kits. If you are traveling or otherwise unable to use standard enema technique, the Fleet's disposable plastic enema outfit works very comfortably and efficiently. By using a special concentrated solution, this outfit gives as much relief from a cupful of material as you would otherwise get from a quart.

Phosphates. If any form of enema is absolutely impractical, an occasional dose of Fleet's Phospho-Soda is probably the most harmless and convenient means of ready relief. One or two teaspoonfuls in a half a glassful of water before breakfast usually give relief by ten a.m. This material has the one drawback that its demands are rather urgent when they arise, so you should not stray too far from facilities.

Rid yourself of constipation worries. Constipation worries are plagues in themselves. Whether you take action against sluggish bowel function or not, take heart from these reassuring facts:

You do not soak up poisons from inside a sluggish bowel. Headache, gas pains, nausea, and other constipation-caused complaints come from pressure on sensitive nerve endings in the rectum. People subject to these complaints are made just as miserable by a rectum packed with cotton as by actual bowel stagnation.

You do not need a movement every day or every other day. Some people average only one movement a week, and still enjoy quiet, comfortable abdomens and soft, easily passed stools. Strive for natural rhythm regulation with good bowel action at your body's own, individually determined interval. Don't try to put your bowel in a time-interval strait jacket.

Small movements may be completely adequate. If a movement passes easily, is of normal consistency, and is not rushed or interrupted, you need not worry about whether it is large enough or not.

Intestinal fermentation simply does not occur. Most stomach and intestinal gas comes from swallowed air. Poisonous gases do not form even if material moves through the intestine very slowly.

SPECIAL FORMS OF CONSTIPATION

A tight bowel occasionally springs from more serious causes than ordinary constipation. Sometimes victims of more serious types of costiveness can get considerable help from home remedies. On other occasions, their awareness of what is going on may lead to better results through prompt doctor care.

Rectal accumulations. An uncomfortable plug of hardened material sometimes accumulates in the rectum. People over sixty who are physically inactive often suffer from this condition. You can usually tell that a plug is accumulating, but straining produces only a little watery discharge. Ordinary enemas give no relief. Severe lower abdominal cramps frequently follow, with loss of appetite, nausea, and sometimes headache.

Oil enemas. You can often get rid of rectal accumulations with simple home measures. The first thing to try is a *slow-action oil enema.* At bedtime, place one cup of warm olive oil in an ordinary enema bag. Use the smallest available tip, and lubricate it well with petroleum jelly. Lie on your left side. Let the oil run in very slowly. Keep your abdomen relaxed. Stop the flow and take several deep breaths through your mouth if you get an urge to expel the oil. When all the oil has run in, withdraw the tip. Lie flat on your back with your buttocks pressed together until you have no further urge to expel the oil, then let it soak in overnight. In the morning, a gentle evacuation often occurs after breakfast. If not, a salt and soda enema is often more effective and more comfortable than it would have been without the oil.

Blocked bowel. Blocked bowel always arises out of some other condition. The vanguards of blocked bowel usually give considerable warning. You can make their cure safer and more comfortable if you get help with them before final blockage occurs.

Hernia is the commonest cause of blocked bowel. It also gives the longest and most easily detected warning. In hernia, organs which belong inside the abdomen slide through a narrow opening in the abdomen's muscle sheath. This happens most commonly in the groin. Sometimes it occurs at or above the navel or within the scar left by a previous operation. If you get a hernia, you will notice a bulging under the skin which shows up more when you strain at stool, or cough. You will not usually have pain, although the stretched muscles in the area may become stiff and sore after you have done heavy work. You may get a sliding or pulling sensation when you cough or strain.

A hernia is dangerous because a length of bowel can slide into it and get stuck. The narrow gap in muscle through which the hernia slides can act just like a noose around your intestine, blocking off the movement of bowel contents. Intestinal obstruction leads to severe cramps all over the abdomen, vomiting, shock, and truly grave illness. If you have any signs of hernia, ward off blocked bowel by seeing your doctor and following his advice. That advice will probably include an operation, but a safe, relatively comfortable one compared with the risks you'll avoid.

The most important other cause of blocked bowel is tumor. A tumor also gives warning, but in less definite ways. Although innocent conditions might well be at fault, you should see your doctor whenever you note any of these signs:

1. Indigestion over a period of three weeks or more.
2. Unexplained weight loss.
3. Abruptly beginning constipation, diarrhea or alternate spells of constipation and diarrhea.
4. Frequent feeling that bowels need to move when an attempt to do so proves futile.

How Harvey Peterson beat his tumor to the punch. When tumor singles out a victim, that person still can win his way back to perfect health. Harvey Peterson's case is a good example. When Harvey first came to my office, he said:

"I've been constipated for the first time in my life these last six weeks. And this morning there was a little blood with my movement. Probably nothing serious, but when you're over forty I guess you can't afford to wait and see."

It's a good thing Harvey felt that way. About a foot from the lower end of his bowel, a tumor surrounded his intestine in a tight, hard band. In a few more weeks or months, that tumor would have blocked the bowel completely, causing painful and dangerous obstruction. But Harvey never suffered that dread state. He had an operation, but not a hurried or extra-hazardous one. Harvey was out of the hospital in ten days and back at work in a month, completely and permanently cured of his disease.

CHAPTER FIVE

How to Heal Rectal and Bladder Complications with Home Measures

There's no misery quite like the misery you get from rectal and bladder troubles, as every sufferer knows. Elimination complaints drag on and on until you think they'll never quit. Most of the commonest ones will yield to simple home measures, though. You can win considerable ease for yourself if you are plagued by hemorrhoids, rectal itching, rectal-opening splits, rectal aftermaths of childbearing or certain bladder ailments.

HOW TO SOOTHE HEMORRHOIDS AT HOME

Home measures can help you to soothe hemorrhoids, to slow their formation or growth, and to make any doctoring they require more comfortable and less expensive. You need surgery for lasting, total cure once hemorrhoids have fully developed, but you can often keep them from reaching that point.

How to soothe clotted hemorrhoids. You can control most discomfort from hemorrhoids with simple home measures. When a hemorrhoid becomes painful, the bulged-out vein inside it usually has become stopped up with a blood clot. This results in swelling, which stretches the sensitive bowel lining or skin. When hemorrhoids hurt, you should try to help your body soak up the clot inside them and try to shrink or soothe the swollen tissue. You can definitely help your body soak up blood clots faster with hot water applied to the painful parts.

Hot towels. Fold an ordinary bath towel until it is six or eight layers thick. Wet it in hot water (about 112 degrees F), and wring it partly dry. Lie face down and place the towel between the buttocks so that it rests against the rectal area. Cover with a dry towel or piece

75

of plastic film to cut down heat loss by evaporation, and dip again as soon as cooling begins. Continue for 20 minutes by the clock.

Hot sitz baths. A frequently more convenient and equally effective method of treating sore hemorrhoids spread through the western world from old-time Germany, where it was known as the "sitzenbad" or sitting bath. Somebody goofed in the course of translation, and the mythical Dr. Sitz has been getting credit for the invention ever since. The technique is simply to sit in about four inches of hot water for exactly 20 minutes. Wrap a towel around your shoulders so that you will not get chilled. Add hot water as required to keep the temperature at 112 degrees. If you do not have an accurate candy or darkroom thermometer, test the water with your hand frequently while heating it up: after your less sensitive parts become accustomed to heat, they sometimes give you no warning even when you add enough hot water to cause a burn. Let a little water out if the depth gets much above four inches: you want to draw more circulation to the sore rectal area, not to the whole surface of your skin.

Irritated hemorrhoids. If hemorrhoids are raw or itchy and not truly painful, try *zinc oxide ointment.* You can get this at your drugstore without prescription. Scoop up a thick glob with an enema tip or with the end of a soft rubber catheter. Insert the instrument gently just into the rectum and withdraw. Apply further ointment to the surface hemorrhoids. A covering film of cotton helps to keep ointment off your clothing.

Suppositories. Wyanoid or Anusol suppositories sometimes help when zinc oxide fails. Unwrap and insert suppositories blunt end first, immediately after each bowel movement.

Increasing or newly formed hemorrhoids You can often make hemorrhoids subside or substantially slow their growth. The effective home measures you can apply for this purpose also improve your rectal comfort. Try this two-pronged attack:

1. Keep veins at the rectal opening from becoming over-engorged. You can often prevent hemorrhoids altogether or markedly slow their growth if you can keep the veins at the rectal opening from becoming over-engorged. Some of the web of veins in this area lead back to the heart through vessels inside the abdomen which branch many times within your liver. Others take a direct route to the heart without going through the abdominal cavity. When you increase the pressure on the veins inside your abdomen by straining at stool, lifting, stooping or coughing, you squeeze blood back from the veins inside the abdomen through the veins near the rectal opening into the free-flowing direct vein passage. Heavy flow of blood under high pressure in the small rectal veins is like heavy truck traffic on a dirt detour; it overloads and damages delicate vein walls.

You can prevent this whole chain of hemorrhoid-forming events by keeping down the pressure within your abdominal cavity. Three approaches are completely practical within your own home:

a. Learn to lift, stoop, and squat without squeezing or grunting. Let open, easy breathing serve as a constant safety valve against built-up abdominal pressures. At first, you will have to train yourself to keep breathing during muscular exertion: deliberately breathe in through your nose and out through your mouth as you lift, squat, stoop, or strain. Later, when this has become a habit, you will find that it not only helps preserve your rectal comfort but also increases your capacity for heavy work.

b. Avoid undue straining at stool. If a movement is very difficult, take a slow-action oil enema (see page 73) instead of proceeding. Follow the constipation control program outlined in Chapter Four for strain-free elimination.

c. Keep effective cough medicine on hand. Even if you could bear up under cough miseries, you can spare your rectum by controlling them.

2. Keep hard passages from aggravating hemorrhoids. When hemorrhoidal veins bulge out, they push the delicate bowel lining or skin into the bowel passage. Bruising and pulling further stretch and irritate the bulged-out tissue. The discomfort of movements leads to spasm, which allows the next movement to get extra hard. Difficult movements lead to pain, spasm, and still more pain: a vicious circle of misery and increasing harm.

If you suffer even slightly from hemorrhoids, you should take steps to keep this vicious circle from making them worse. The constipation cure from Chapter Four is very much worthwhile, but hemorrhoid sufferers should take these extra steps:

1. Get a soft rubber catheter, size 24 or 28, from your drugstore or surgical supply house. Use it in place of the usual hard rubber tip whenever you need an enema. Use lubricating jelly instead of petroleum jelly on the catheter, since petroleum jelly rots rubber. Insert only an inch or two for ordinary enemas, up to six or eight inches for oil.

2. Instill one ounce of olive or mineral oil into the rectum at bedtime whenever no bowel movement has occurred for two or more days. An all rubber ear syringe, which you can get at any drugstore for about a dollar, makes this procedure very easy and comfortable.

3. Take plain Metamucil or a similar moist-bulk providing agent regularly in doses large enough to produce at least one movement every two days, if natural rhythm regulation makes for less frequent stools.

Protruding hemorrhoids. If a too-firm bowel movement pulls hemorrhoids from inside the rectal opening, you should slide them back in place promptly. Smooth pressure through several layers of toilet paper may do the trick. Lubricate the hemorrhoids with olive or mineral oil on a cotton ball if necessary. When discomfort is considerable, the muscle which cuts off the flow of bowel discharges has become tight around the hemorrhoids. Soothe the area with several minutes of hot applications for easier replacement of the protruding piles. Hot, wet towels or sitting in four inches of hot water works quite well.

When your doctor's help is worthwhile for hemorrhoids. If you have hemorrhoids, you usually need a doctor's help to prove that you have no serious underlying conditon. You often need his help to achieve a complete and lasting cure.

Anything which causes enlargement or change in an abdominal organ, from pregnancy or ovarian cyst to rectal cancer or liver disease, can cause detouring of blood through the veins at the rectal opening and make hemorrhoids form. If hemorrhoids bleed in such a way that blood mixes in through the stool instead of merely showing on the paper, or if there are other signs of internal disorder such as change in bowel habit, weight loss, or pencil-shaped, small stools, you have an excellent chance of stopping a serious disorder, before it gets a foothold, by seeing your doctor promptly. You can usually put off examination for hemorrhoids that only bleed on the paper until your next visit to a doctor for some other complaint. Ask for a complete rectal examination at that time: your doctor can usually tell without putting you to any extra expense or inconvenience whether any underlying problem is present.

Injection treatments or operation usually gives complete and permanent cure for hemorrhoids. If all your hemorrhoids originate inside the rectal opening, when you see your doctor you can usually avoid operation altogether. At this stage, internal hemorrhoids yield to painless injection treatments done in your doctor's office instead of in the hospital. If your condition does call for operation, though, don't let old wive's tales frighten you: today's methods of pain relief and gentleness will positively keep you from suffering severe discomfort.

Sore hemorrhoids as large as or larger than the tip of your thumb or hemorrhoids which fail to subside with heat and ointment deserve the prompt relief your doctor can give.

HOW TO RELIEVE RECTAL ITCHING

The secret of curing ordinary rectal itching, whether you have hemorrhoids or not, is to soothe the irritation caused by material which seeps out from the bowel. After each bowel movement, take these four steps:

1. Cleanse the rectal area with soap and warm water on a soft washrag. Follow with several spongings of plain water to rinse away the soap. This procedure is much less irritating than rubbing raw, scratch-scored skin with any kind of paper, even facial tissue.

2. Sponge off entire area with rubbing alcohol. This kills germs and helps dry the macerated skin.

3. Powder the area with talc or cornstarch. A drying powder helps the skin to resist itch-producing fluids which seep out of the rectum.

4. Take a wisp of cotton about half as big as a cigarette, powder it with talc or cornstarch, smooth it over the tip of your index finger and insert it about half an inch into the rectal opening, just far enough so that it will stay in place. This acts as a wick to prevent seepage. If large hemorrhoids are present, you may need to make the piece of cotton somewhat larger and put it a bit farther into the opening to keep it in place.

How to cure rectal dermatitis at home. If rectal itching is severe and application of rubbing alcohol burns or stings badly, your case has probably reached the stage of rectal dermatitis. Apply cloths wet with Burow's solution three or four times a day for ten minutes. You can get either tablets or concentrate with which to make Burow's solution from your druggist without a prescription. Use one tablet or one tablespoonful of concentrate to a pint of lukewarm water. After two to four days of applying Burow's you can usually switch to the alcohol-talc-wick method used for ordinary itching.

Malt soup extract. A few victims of rectal itching or dermatitis find that they can rid themselves of this misery altogether with malt soup extract. You will find this material at the infant feeding section of your drugstore instead of in with the medicines. Take one tablespoonful either mixed with cereal or stirred in water with each of your three meals.

When your doctor can help with rectal itching. Your doctor can give worthwhile aid for rectal itching under several different circumstances:

1. Rectal itching after bedtime often means pinworms, especially

in households with preschool and early-grade youngsters. About one-third of children in this age group have pinworms. Adults in their families often become involved. Fortunately, piperazine (antepar) cures most cases permanently without the mess and bother of enemas and other measures which old-fashioned treatment usually required.

2. Persistent cases get relief with hydrocortisone ointment and other prescription-only products.

3. Rectal itching associated with pain, discomfort, or bulging usually is due to some underlying condition such as split at the bowel opening or hemorrhoids. The underlying disorder may need medical treatment before you get relief.

PINWORMS

I'll stack Minnesota households against any in the world for cleanliness. Yet I've seen as many as forty per cent of the youngsters in a Minnesota kindergarten prove to have pinworms. In fact, I've gotten to the point where any preschool youngster in my office who squirms and pulls at clothing in his body creases gets a test for this condition immediately. Squirming and restlessness are easier to spot than itching—youngsters often don't zero in on discomforts precisely and may not really "scratch where it itches"—but scratching around the seat or vaginal irritation may also point to pinworm problems.

Home check for pinworms. When your youngsters are in their soundest sleep, usually between eleven and twelve at night, mother pinworm crawls out of the rectum and lays her eggs. This is the source of all that later itching, squirming and discomfort—and you can catch her at her work if you just look. You'll find that you can expose the rectal area and look very thoroughly without even rousing your sleeping preschooler (or early-elementary-schooler). If present, the worms look like little bits of white thread about half an inch in length. They will often be in folds and creases, so you will need to spread the skin slightly in different directions in order to spot them. Use a bright flashlight for further aid.

Doctor tests for pinworms. Your doctor can't tell whether or not pinworms are present by examining a specimen of stool. The easiest way with youngsters is to stick some Scotch tape over the rectal area, peel it off, and examine it under the microscope. When growth of hair makes this test impractical, gentle skin scrapings work best.

Treatment. Pinworms build up by vicious-circle action. Eggs laid on the skin cause itching, scratching gets eggs on the hands and from there they get back into the mouth either on food or through thumb-sucking, etc. You can clear up the problem over a long period of time by keeping the child's fingernails trimmed down close and keeping him or her clothed (especially at night) in a way which makes it impossible to scratch.

For quick results, though, there are no home measures to match prescription ones. The usual prescription remedy (piperazine) is both highly effective and free of unpleasant side effects. One problem: pinworm eggs in their dry form float all over the house and usually affect everyone in it to some degree. If you go the quick, medicinal route, best treat everyone in the family at once (including the adults) to keep the untreated ones from reinfecting the rest.

RECTAL SPLITS AND FISSURES

You can almost always cure the commonest painful condition at the rectal opening for yourself in your own home and avoid the need for rectal surgery if you take action promptly. A split in the surface layer of the rectal opening causes considerable discomfort. Your first warning is often a tearing sensation followed by burning pain, which occurs during the passage of a hard stool. In other cases, pain may increase gradually, usually beginning at the conclusion of a move-ment and lasting 30 seconds to five minutes. After the onset of the rectal split, movements cause some burning discomfort during the passage of stool and red-hot-poker pain immediately thereafter. Since any form of rectal pain usually tightens the bowel, constipation aggravates the problem.

Severe discomfort after bowel movements almost always means a rectal split. Take these steps promptly for surgery-saving home cure:

1. Assure soft, easily passed movements while the rectal split heals. Take a teaspoonful of *Metamucil* twice daily, mixing each with one glass of water and following with another. Get a two-ounce all-rubber ear syringe. Fill it with *olive or mineral* oil. At bedtime, insert the soft rubber tip just inside the rectum. Slowly squeeze the oil into the bowel cavity. Withdraw the syringe, and put a sanitary pad (as Kotex) or pad of cotton in place to catch any oil which seeps out during the night. Use full-sized, six ounce slow action oil enemas (see page 73) at night if movements do not occur daily, and follow with a *salt and soda enema* given through a soft rubber catheter rather than an ordinary enema tip if no movement has occurred by 10 o'clock the next morning (see pages 66-67).

2. Soothe the split at the rectal opening. Put a glob of *zinc oxide ointment* on the tip of the ear syringe when you take your nightly stool-softening treatment. Apply zinc oxide ointment in a similar way twice during the day. If the split is very sore, use Surfacaine ointment or Nupercainal for a few days instead of zinc oxide.

3. Relieve spasm in the muscle which cuts off the flow of bowel contents. Use soothing heat three times a day by applying *hot wet towels* or sitz baths. If pain or muscle spasm persists, use astringent or antispasmodic (Anusol or Wyanoid) suppositories every 12 hours Unwrap and insert each suppository blunt end first.

This home program for healing rectal splits will almost always do the trick inside four weeks. If a rectal split already has a head start or fails to respond to home measures, your doctor can heal it for you with surgery. The operation required is not an unusually painful one. It can sometimes be done without hospitalization, and never requires more than a day or two of hospital care.

HOME MEASURES A WOMAN CAN USE FOR CYSTOCOEL AND RECTOCOEL

You can often prevent or control by prompt action the two commonest special female problems of elimination which otherwise lead to years of nagging discomfort, and often to ultimate surgery. These conditions arise through bulging of the rectum or the bladder into the female organ. Rectocoel or cystocoel usually plagues women whose tissues have been stretched in childbirth, although childless women are not immune. Both conditions are usually present in severe cases.

How to control rectocoel or cystocoel. Proper elimination keeps down strain on the thin walls of tissue which separate the rectum and bladder from the female opening. Even if you already suffer from slipping and sliding sensations or slight bulging, these steps may keep rectocoel and cystocoel under control:

1. Prevent bulge-forming abdominal pressures by controlling constipation and severe cough. Follow the program for constipation outlined in Chapter Four. Get prescription-strength (½ grain of codeine per dose) cough syrup from your doctor when you get a severe cold.

2. Heed nature's calls. An over-full bladder presses down and stretches the wall between it and the vagina. A bowel movement which has become difficult through unwarranted delay places strain on the tissues which divide the rectum from the female canal. You can avoid both unnecessary strains by heeding nature's calls promptly.

3. Empty your bowels in a posture which directs the advancing stool directly out the rectum opening or to the rear of it. When you sit upright with your feet flat on the floor, the advancing stool drives into the wall between rectum and vagina. This flimsy wall must turn it toward the proper opening. The least tendency to be swaybacked increases this problem tremendously: arch the lower portion of your back forward, and you will see how hollow-backed posture directs material from the abdomen toward the front of the elimination tube. You can correct these problems in three easy ways: You can roll your pelvis forward as you sit, as if you were trying to look at the female opening during the movement. You can increase the bend of your knees and the fold of your hips by putting your feet on a high footstool and leaning well forward or by clasping your arms around your knees during actions. Or you can learn to squat on the toilet rim with the seat up, which directs the advancing stool properly in almost every single case.

One of my patients, for instance, complained that she could not expel a bowel movement except by pressing her fingers against the back of her vagina. When she assumed her usual sway-backed sitting posture, the reason was all too clear: material moving down her rectum had to turn nearly a right angle on its way to the outer opening. The flimsy recto-vaginal wall was not strong enough to deflect firm movements, so a tremendous forward bulge had formed. Surgery was the only answer by that time, but the whole chain of events could have been prevented or ameliorated if she had only learned to empty her bowels in a flexed posture some years before.

4. Strengthen separations between various openings with pelvic exercises. Any woman who has had a child should build the strength of her pelvic muscles. You can do pelvic exercises either sitting up or lying down, in the privacy of your own home or while you are riding on the bus to work: wherever you have a few moments undisturbed. First, try to squeeze the female opening together with its own musculature, as if you were picking up marbles with it. Hold the muscles contracted for three to five seconds, then relax. Next, try to lift the bowel opening straight up into the pelvis. Hold it for three to five seconds, then relax. Continue alternating these two kinds of contraction of pelvic musculature for about two minutes. Follow this routine three times a day for three to four weeks to build pelvic muscle strength, then once a day to maintain it. (This same exercise greatly increases your capacity to satisfy your husband sexually. Not only does it make for snugger union, but it teaches voluntary control. After you get the muscles built up, try pumping them

rapidly in this same order during sexual relations, or squeezing and relaxing the vagina at the sex climax. Your husband will love you for it!)

5. Drink plenty of extra water. Besides bulging discomforts, cystocoel frequently causes bladder irritation. This causes you to have to urinate frequently, often with little advance notice or urge. Burning discomfort on urination may also plague you. You can usually stave off this kind of trouble by keeping the urinary passages flushed out with copious urinary flow. Two to three quarts of water, fruit juice or non-cola containing beverages usually does the trick.

When your doctor can give worthwhile help with rectocoel and cystocoel. Your doctor can usually arrange relief for you if you suffer from rectocoel or cystocoel. Sometimes a supporting internal brace helps. In more severe cases, operation gives fairly thorough relief. Surgery is quite safe and does not keep you inactive for very long.

HOME CARE FOR CYSTITIS

The shortness and breadth of the tube from the bladder to the exterior makes women particularly subject to cystitis, although some men suffer from it, too. Attacks usually start with burning and stinging on urination. The urge to void becomes frequent, sometimes every five minutes. Victims often complain that they still feel an unrequited urge after voiding. Urine usually looks cloudy or smoky, and sometimes appears bloody, too. This condition may cause one or two degrees of fever.

Home care for early and mild cystitis. The germs which start a bladder infection often die out if you change the chemical character of your urine through simple home measures. This is particularly true at the very beginning of infection, when very few germs have had a chance to burrow into the bladder wall and virtually all are still bathed in urine. Take these two steps at the very first sign of burning, frequent urination, or a sense of being unable to empty the bladder:

1. Drink copious amounts of water, ginger ale, orange juice, or lemonade. Try to down at least three or four extra quarts of fluid each day. You'll find you can drink more by taking a small juice glass every 10 or 15 minutes than by trying to choke down a whole glassful every hour. Moderately chilled drinks usually pass through the stomach more quickly than ice cold ones, too.

2. Take two teaspoonfuls of baking soda in a little water every

two hours during waking hours for two or three days, provided you have no heart or kidney trouble. Do not take this step if your doctor has told you to avoid excess salt: the sodium ion, which is what he wants you to avoid, is contained in baking soda as well as table salt.

Spasm soothing suppositories. Wyanoids suppositories or medically prescribed spasm soothers often give considerable relief from cystitis. They do not speed your cure particularly, but they relieve discomfort and allow a longer interval between voidings.

How to ward off toilet paper cystitis. Germs often get a big head start in moving from the intestinal opening to the bladder by faulty cleansing technique. You can carry a positive horde of cystitis-causing germs forward to the urinary outlet with one forward stroke of the toilet paper. This very common source of bladder infection is easy to dodge: simply avoid reaching between your legs to cleanse your rectal opening, keeping your cleaning motions to the rectal area itself instead of including the genital zone, and use each tissue for only one front-to-back stroke.

Honeymoon cystitis. Another common aid to cystitis germs on their passage up the urinary tract is sexual activity. Intercourse in positions where the man's angle of entrance directs the penis toward the front of the vagina catches the urinary tube against the inside of the pelvic bones and milks germs along it. Although these positions give great satisfaction at times, they predispose toward cystitis during periods of very frequent intercourse, such as a honeymoon or reunion after a long absence.

Sex position during highly active periods. Whenever you expect to have relations more than three times a week, you should avoid sex postures in which the man's angle of entrance brings the penis snugly against the front wall of the vagina. The only two common postures in which this occurs are the folded hip postures, in which the woman folds her hips after entry and either hooks her heels on her husband's shoulders or pulls her knees up close to her armpits. The standard position and woman's-legs-down-straight position put absolutely no strain on the bladder, and can be used freely during frequent-sex periods.

Drink plenty of water. Adequate flow of urine helps to flush away any germs that get close to your bladder. If you heed your body's thirst signals, this need is ordinarily met. I have seen several women who developed bladder infections after cutting down on liquids at and after supper in order to avoid getting up at night to urinate. Certainly, such limitation is most unwise during lively-sex weeks.

When your doctor can give worthwhile help with cystitis. Thanks to today's large assortment of powerful germ killing medicines, your doctor can almost always cure cystitis in a matter of hours. You don't need to suffer along for days if home measures fail to help you.

Even if home measures are effective against cystitis, your doctor's help is worthwhile in two instances:

When you have passed blood in your urine, special examinations are necessary. Many of the urinary disorders whose first warning is bloody urine yield much more readily to prompt than to delayed treatment. Since these conditions may mimic bladder infection quite closely, anyone who passes blood should have a complete examination of the bladder and kidneys.

A man who has two attacks or a woman who has three attacks of cystitis should have special examinations to search for a smoldering source of infection or an abnormality which makes him especially liable to urinary disease. This examination should at least include special kidney X-rays, and usually also an examination of the inside of the bladder. Doctors can identify and cure almost all of the conditions which lead to repeated urinary infections at this stage, whereas they might not be able to do so later.

Bedwetting. "I don't know what we're going to do with George," Clarice said, shooing her ten-year-old toward my examining table. "He's scheduled to go to church camp next month, and he's still wetting the bed."

Attempting to shame a youngster out of bedwetting often backs the whole family into a corner. My heart went out to young George, who obviously wished he could find a crack to crawl into. But at this point he needed something more than sympathy.

"Does he have to strain for a long time to get the stream started when he urinates?" I asked. "Some youngsters have a flap of tissue or a constriction in the tube out from the bladder and have a hard time emptying their bladders. The stagnation causes smoldering infection, and that makes them wet the bed."

"I hadn't even thought of anything like that," Clarice said.

"Then there are the sound sleepers," I went on. "Boys who just don't wake up until after it's too late. We can usually help them get over bedwetting pretty easily, and of course it isn't their fault that they sleep soundly."

"George sleeps like a rock, all right. In fact, even when you get him up and walk him to the bathroom, he doesn't remember a thing about it in the morning."

"Let's try the conditioned reflex system for a little while, then, and see whether we can tie the act of voiding a little more tightly to the bathroom."

When the Russian scientist Pavlov rang a bell each time he fed his dogs, he found later that he could make them slobber just by ringing the bell. You can use the same action as a training aid, although I think it is more pleasant to use a little music box rather than a bell. If the child turns on a music box every time he gets ready to void in the daytime, he will link that sound and the bathroom surroundings with the act of urination. After a few weeks of this, he will have sound, spot and action linked together in his mind. If you get him up just before you go to bed, take him to the bathroom, and start the music box playing, he will usually void quite readily. After a few weeks of nightly emptying, he will often reach a point where he gets up without aid instead of wetting the bed.

CHAPTER SIX

Home Remedies for Sexual
and Menopausal Complaints

Sexual afflictions are triply disturbing. They make you miserable, they frequently lead to embarrassment, and they undermine your sexual self-confidence. Why suffer messy discharge, embarrassing itch, sexually debilitating congestion, and menopausal miseries? Home care can help you with all of these conditions and many others.

HOW TO CONTROL FEMALE TROUBLES
WITH HOME MEASURES

Mild or moderate discharge, itching, and irritation of the female outlet frequently yield to simple home measures. Profuse watery discharge usually deserves a doctor's care, especially if it causes a great deal of itching, burning or surface rawness. So does thick, whitish discharge accompanied by severe itching which is often due to fungus infection. Women in their sixties and seventies often suffer from a special form of vaginal irritation and discharge which yields promptly to female sex hormones, and often get worthwhile help from a doctor. If you decide that prescription measures might help you, always take a sanitary belt and several pads to the doctor's office with you, since some of the medicines used stain clothing irreparably.

Whitish discharge. Ordinary whitish discharge usually yields to vinegar douching, which you can manage quite well at home.

Vinegar douches. Plain vinegar restores vaginal acidity and clears up most cases of simple discharge. Use an ordinary douche bag with a hard rubber tip. Make up the douche solution with four tablespoonfuls of white vinegar and two quarts of warm water. Lubricate the douche tip with petroleum or lubricating jelly, and insert it. Hold the lips of the female organ snugly together around the base of the tip, and start the solution running in with the bag a foot or two above the douche tip opening. When water pressure balloons out the organ and opens up all the deep wrinkles and creases, you will feel a slight stretching sensation. Release the lips of the female organ and let the douche fluid flow freely for a moment while the vagina collapses into folds again. Repeat this process several times, until the douche fluid is exhausted. Most victims of ordinary discharge need to douche daily for about ten days and two to three times weekly thereafter.

How to control itching at the female opening. Itching of the female opening without excessive discharge often yields to home measures. Try this program:

First two days: Cleanse the area twice daily with a mild detergent such as pHisoderm and several cotton balls. Four times daily, mix one tablespoonful of Burow's solution with one cup of water and use to wet a washcloth or piece of cotton. Place this against the itching area for ten minutes.

Until itching is completely controlled (usually about one week): Get one ounce of Lassar's paste from your druggist (no prescription required). Dry thoroughly after each cleansing and apply a thin coat of the paste.

After itching ceases: Continue cleansing once a day. Dry thoroughly. Powder lightly with cornstarch. Continue this program for two weeks.

Your doctor can give worthwhile help if itching does not yield promptly to this program or if it is accompanied by excessive discharge, a lump, or a sore or leathery white patch.

HOME MANAGEMENT OF MASTURBATION

"I just know he's playing with himself," Gloria said. "I'll find stiff soiled handkerchiefs around, and sometimes dirty pictures. But he doesn't have a father, you know, and I just can't bring myself to talk about it."

Gloria's son was a well-developed fifteen, old enough to have sired a child or two when humankind hid out in caves and bushes, but still a mere boy according to our present lights. Hormones change a few eons less quickly than civilization's customs, though, and the boy had all the glandular functions of a grown and married man.

"I'll talk to him if you want," I said. "But I'm probably not going to say what you expect."

Reassurance. "I'll tell him just what my old professor used to say: ninety percent of boys admit to masturbation and the other ten per cent are liars. I know that some churches regard it as a sin, and I'll make it clear to him that the rights and wrongs of masturbation aren't entirely based on medical facts. But I'll try to set him straight on any old wives' tales he's heard about masturbation stunting his growth or affecting his mind and any confusion he might have of masturbation and homosexuality."

We had our little talk a few days later, but I'm not sure it made very much difference. The main problem was Gloria's undue concern, which was relieved long before I saw her son.

Masturbation injury. Physical injury from masturbation is not a problem with boys, but girls (over half of whom also use some form of sexual self-stimulation) sometimes have difficulties. When a girl complains of whitish, irritating discharge, she often has a small object or a piece of an object up inside the vagina. If you can approach the subject in a way which does not seem harshly critical or accusatory, she will often tell you what has happened. In most cases, these objects can readily be removed without medical instruments. Bleeding sometimes comes from a torn virginal membrane. If you spread the folds so that you can see where the bleeder is spurting, firm pressure with a cotton ball for five minutes by the clock (without any interruption for peeks to see whether the treatment is working) will usually stop the flow. In these situations, and also in those requiring medical care, it is important to approach the problem in a matter-of-fact, noncritical manner—shame and embarrassment are great strains to the young mind, and often interfere with later sexual adjustment. Why add these burdens to the already substantial adjustment problems of youth?

Undue sexual curiosity. Many years ago, a six-year-old boy was brought to me because he "took down the neighbor's young girl's panties."

"It's natural and normal for a six-year-old to want to know more about the difference between boys and girls," I said. "He could probably have picked a way that wouldn't offend neighborhood manners and morals, but there's nothing wrong with his mind or his sexual development."

"Then we shouldn't do anything about it?" the boy's parents asked.

"Have a little talk with him, if you can do it without getting embarrassed or upset, but aim at assuaging his curiosity instead of condemning his behavior. Show him pictures, explain how the male and female organs fit together. If you can feel totally comfortable about it, you might let down the modesty barriers a bit around the house—our household works on the assumption that the sight of your private parts is something which should be reserved for members of the family, but needn't be restricted particularly within that circle. We went that route mainly for the sake of the girls—I've seen too many women who had trouble adjusting to marriage mainly because they were embarrassed about being seen—but it's a good way to avoid pent-up curiosity, too."

I dug back into ancient history for this case because I know how that youngster turned out: he's a respected minister, happily married and father of three children. He has never been involved in any sexual impropriety since, in spite of (or more likely because of) his parents' tolerant, noncritical response to this incident.

HOW TO CONTROL COMMON MALE SEX MISERIES WITH HOME MEASURES

You can avoid or quickly cure penile irritations, urethritis, and some prostate troubles with home measures. Cleansing methods, contraceptive or hygienic measures, sex habits, and fluid balance all enter into your program for controlling sex organ difficulties. Medicines and special supplies are seldom required.

Crab lice. Most victims pick up crab lice from public toilets, not by sex contact. Look for the little devils whenever you get much itching down below. They are brownish in color and almost half as big as an ordinary wood tick. Sometimes you can spot the pearly gray eggs adhering to pubic hairs more easily than the burrowing lice.

Ointment. I usually suggest Kwell ointment for crab lice. Apply to the crotch, pubic hair area, and armpits twice a day for two days.

DDT. Ten per cent DDT powder is cheaper than ointment, and is quite effective in most cases. Apply two or three times a day for three days.

Shave, trim or comb. With DDT powder and other methods aimed at the adult lice only, you need to shave the whole area gently but thoroughly or go over it with a fine toothed comb. The fine toothed comb works best if you have applied towels wet with vinegar solution (two tablespoonfuls to a pint of warm water) for 20 minutes. Since the recommended ointment kills eggs as well as lice, you can trim the hairs to half inch length with this method instead or shaving or combing, and avoid considerable discomfort.

Laundry precautions. Home laundry or helpy-selfy machines do not use hot enough water to kill out crabs. Best send underclothing to a commercial laundry or boil it for ten minutes.

Crotch itch. Another common condition spread through locker room benches and the like is crotch or jock-strap itch. This is a distant cousin of athlete's foot, caused by the same family of microbes. It shows up as dusky red patches on the inner sides of both upper thighs, sometimes with slight scaling. Undecenylic acid ointment (Desenex) twice a day for a week usually affects a cure.

Penile irritations. A sore on the penis within eight weeks after somewhat random sexual contact deserves prompt medical care. Likewise any sore or lump which does not heal promptly with home measures. However, most penile irritations yield quickly to simple home care.

Smegma irritation. Instead of ordinary skin oil, the glands inside the foreskin make a thick, smelly, whitish material. When the tip of the penis or foreskin becomes raw, irritation from this smegma is often at fault.

Thorough cleansing. Smegma irritation usually clears up promptly if you cleanse thoroughly beneath the foreskin every day for a week. Prevent recurrences by cleansing once a week. During a warm bath, strip back the foreskin and wash away any accumulated whitish matter. If the foreskin is tight, be sure to pull it forward again immediately after cleansing: otherwise, the squeeze it makes on the penis may cause enough swelling to make replacement painful or difficult.

Glycerin. A few men find that their smegma is particularly difficult to remove with soap and water. They get relief with a little glycerin applied with cotton, then wiped off five to ten minutes later with a washrag or clean cloth.

Irritation after intercourse. Itchy, burning swellings of the penis within 24 hours after intercourse are usually due to contraceptive or feminine hygiene preparations which your wife is using. A change in brands of birth control materials and replacement of fancy douche powders with ordinary vinegar usually gives quick cure.

Occasionally, I see a patient with swelling and soreness on the under side of the tip of the penis, where a slim band of tissue attaches the foreskin to the head of the penis itself. This almost always stems from excessive sexual friction. Lubrication with lubricating or petroleum jelly during sexual relations usually prevents further difficulty, and aids sexual satisfaction, too.

Irritation from harsh chemicals. Itching and rash on the shaft of the penis usually is due to chemicals or irritants you handle or get on your clothing during the day, transferred to the penis during urination. Cutting oils and chemicals which will not irritate the thick skin of your fingers often make the delicate skin of the penis raw. Solution: Wash your hands thoroughly before urinating, and drop soiled work trousers instead of using the fly. If this fails (as with one of my patients, who ultimately proved allergic to the soap supplied at his working place!), handle the organ through several layers of a clean handkerchief when you need to void during working hours.

How to control urethritis. Although any whitish discharge or burning on urination should send you to your doctor immediately if you have had sexual contact with a possibly infected woman inside two weeks, many infections of the urethra occur without any possibility of venereal disease. In these cases, prompt home measures at the first sign of burning or discharge often lead to cure.

Flooding with fluid. If you drink four to five quarts of water, ginger ale, or fruit juice a day for two to three days starting immediately after the first twinge of burning, you can frequently flush out the urethra thoroughly enough to control the attack.

After-sex urination. If you are subject to nonvenereal infection of the tube from the bladder to the exterior, empty your bladder soon after intercourse. This condition commonly occurs when the germs from the body surface manage to get up into the more delicate portions of the urethra. These germs cannot grow in or swim along the fast-moving urinary stream, but they can grow along or swim up through the protein-rich moisture left behind by sexual excitement or intercourse. Prompt urination usually washes away any residue of protein-rich fluid before germs have a chance to multiply in it and cause an infection.

What about "morning pearl"? After a long period of abstinence from sex, many men begin to find a drop or two of thick white matter at the penile opening every morning. This so-called morning pearl is usually due to very mild non-venereal infection or to simple overflow of sex gland secretion. If sexual relief is not possible, flushing the passage by means of high fluid intake usually brings relief.

Prostate congestion. Impaired potency, low backache and tiredness usually point toward congestion or infection of the prostate gland. While severe cases call for a doctor's care, you can often restore potency and gain comfort in mild cases with home measures.

Hot sitz baths. Put four inches of hot water (112 degrees) in your bathtub. Sit in it for 20 minutes, adding more hot water as necessary to maintain the temperature. If you do not have an accurate thermometer, test the water with your hand when adding hot water to insure against burns. Wrap a towel around your shoulders during the sitz bath to keep from getting chilled.

Scrotal dip. Although hot sitz baths often help to relieve the congestion that leads to sagging potency, the heat tends to soothe sexual excitement to a degree. If you plan prompt sexual exercise, you may find a ten to thirty second dip of the scrotal contents in very cold water helpful. Ice water in an ordinary tumbler works quite well in restoring excitability.

Prostate infection. You usually get worthwhile help from your doctor if you are suffering from actual prostate infection. Extreme impairment of potency, backache, burning on urination, and some-times slight discharge point toward this condition. One helpful home test is the three-glass procedure: pass a few drops of urine in one glass, almost all of what remains in another glass, and the last teaspoonful in a third. Cloudiness in the first glass only usually points to urethritis, while cloudiness in both the first and the third glass almost always means prostate infection.

Prostate disorder proneness. If you have had several spells of prostatitis or if you have smoldering, nonvenereal urethritis, you should rigorously avoid jolting and vibration. A rough ride in a truck or tractor milks material in and out of the prostate gland. If any germs have worked their way back along the urethra to the prostate's opening, which is just below the bladder, the prostate gland becomes infected. The steps we already discussed for avoiding urethritis obviously help to keep germs away from the prostate opening, and thus make jolting and vibration less dangerous. A hydraulic seat or several layers of foam rubber padding help to make vibrating machinery, trucks or tractors less hazardous. A high intake of fluids during working hours makes for more frequent voiding, which flushes germs away from the prostate opening.

Prostate enlargement. When the prostate gland enlarges, it pushes up into the tube from the bladder to the outside. While the prostate seldom blocks the urethra completely, it often prevents the bladder from entirely emptying itself. When your prostate gland enlarges, you may notice some difficulty in starting to urinate. The urinary stream may become less forceful. A sense of not completely emptying the bladder is common. Since the bladder does not empty completely, it fills again more quickly than before: frequent voiding during the day and two or more trips to the toilet at night become necessary. If the condition gets no care, infection usually occurs, causing burning, fever, and extreme frequency. The enlarged gland may block the urinary passage entirely, making the bladder expand painfully.

Hot packs. As a temporary measure of relief, you can often get the urinary stream started by applying hot towels to the crotch and lower abdomen. Change the towels frequently. Usually, it is wise to let a small stream of water run from the tap, too: the sound of running water often helps to relieve tension in the urinary muscles.

Whenever prostate enlargement makes special measures necessary to start the stream, you can definitely get worthwhile help from your doctor. Most such trouble is due to a disorder which never causes cancer. Your doctor can arrange to have the portion of the gland which is blocking the urinary passage pared back electrically, thus avoiding all need for a cutting operation.

HOW TO EASE YOUR WAY THROUGH THE MENOPAUSE

The menopause! How often have you heard that word uttered with a fearful shudder? Until modern science learned to prevent or relieve them, many people suffered grave distress from the miseries of the menopause. Sex organs became a source of botheration and distress to most women and to many men. Today, you can prevent or quickly cure every affliction the menopause might bring. You can keep your sex life satisfying for many years beyond. You can solve most menopause-period sex problems for yourself, right in your own home.

About half of the women and one-fourth of the men in America need help from a doctor for menopausal complaints at one time or another. The problems which yield most readily to prescription-type hormones are hot flashes, sinking spells, abrupt sweating spells, periods of mental fogginess, and creeping, crawling skin sensations. If you suffer from such complaints, a few tablets usually give tremendous help. There is no need to hold back because of fear that you will become more needful of hormones because of what you take. Hormone tablets work to cushion the shock of abrupt change in your body's natural hormone levels. You can usually cut your dose in half within six months and taper to no tablets at all within two years.

Incidentally, tablets work just as well as shots. Thousands of men and women pay needlessly large sums for help with the menopause because of the unwarranted idea that shots are better than pills. The hormone gets into your bloodstream before it has any effect, and it gets there just as reliably from your stomach as from your hip.

Fight menopausal blues with this philosophy. Most of my patients have found one measure even more helpful than hormones in fighting menopausal miseries: developing a different viewpoint toward this period of life. The menopause is not the end of something. It is the beginning of your period of reward: the period when the effort you have put into raising a family begins to justify itself in their success, when your skills and interests bear top fruit, when the home you struggled to build up and keep is all your own. Nothing stops with the menopause, except the inconvenience of monthly bleeding. Sex continues, love continues, strength and skill remain unchanged. That simple fact affords tremendous relief from the blue feelings many people name as the menopause's most stringent plague.

How to enjoy sex after the menopause. A great many women are surprised to find that sex either remains just as enjoyable or even becomes considerably more so after the menopause. Until the menopause, the possibility of pregnancy hangs heavily over every couple's sex life. A woman is never unconcerned about fertility: either she wants babies or she doesn't. She can't indulge in sex for love and pleasure alone as long as pregnancy might possibly result.

After the menopause, neither *hope for* nor *fear of* pregnancy interferes. Both husband and wife can cast off many grave concerns and uncertainties. Each can pursue sex for his own and his partner's satisfaction with concentration and skill never before possible.

How to develop your sexual skill. Selfish sex is always a failure. That's why sexual skill always aims at satisfying the other person. Your partner's response then increases your pleasure and satisfaction. Here are three pointers about married sex which most couples find worthwhile:

Preen for your partner. By age thirty-five or so, many husbands and wives unwittingly begin to take their marriage partners for granted sexually. They pass up simple ways of making themselves more attractive. They don't take time to preen. A little more effort devoted to evening showers, shaves, toothbrushing, perfume, negligee and other bedtime grooming (not to mention negatives like face cream, curlers and such) often makes more difference than the best-planned erotic campaign.

Keep variety in your caresses. It's wonderful to know what your sex partner likes, and to put that knowledge to work. But if you could sit down right now and write the exact caresses your husband or wife will expect the next time you have sex, variety could add new heights of excitement to your marriage bed. Change the order of your approach. Change the type of caress from stroke to grasp, from kiss to gentle nip, from rhythmic rub to vibrating tickle. Give special care to the last stage of your sex play: full passionate preparation calls for culminating caresses which should never seem routine.

Gain new thrills or greater ease and comfort through different sex positions. A husband and wife can fit together sexually in literally dozens of ways. The standard position has one advantage: both husband and wife can contribute what they wish with caresses, loving words, and activity. Certain other positions help keep your sexual attraction ever fresh by adding variety. Still others meet certain frequent health or sexual needs. Here are the most important special approaches:

Important nerve centers come into play with the wife in a bent-knees, bent hips posture, especially after you reach full-blown maturity. Through the years of marriage, sex sensitivity gradually shifts in the female organ. Spots toward the front far up inside the female organ become keener. The husband can often please and satisfy a mature wife much more thoroughly if he directs his thrust forward. To do this, he brings his wife's knees up beside his chest with her hips folded.

Any long-married couple can vary their sex life through the wife's-heels-on-husband's shoulders position. They begin intercourse in standard position. After contact, the wife stretches her legs straight up. The husband rears back slightly, and moves his arms one at a time to a position outside his wife's legs. The wife then hooks the back of her heels on his shoulders. The husband contributes all sexual activity from then on, although his wife can respond freely with words and caresses.

Make your union snugger with the wife's-legs-straight position. A woman who has borne several children may have a stretched, over-spacious vagina. This makes it hard for her to satisfy her husband. But if she keeps her legs straight down and her husband spreads his legs to straddle hers, both partners can reach a keen climax.

Enjoy sex without exertion with the postero-lateral or the crossed approach. Both these positions allow moderate sexual satisfaction when illness or loss of strength makes vigorous approach difficult. For the postero-lateral approach, both partners lie on their right sides. The husband approaches from the rear while the wife keeps her hips and knees bent. The crossed position finds the wife lying on her back with hips folded. The husband lies on his right side crosswise on the bed.

CHAPTER SEVEN

Home Remedies for Colds, Sore Throats, and Coughs

Of all the miseries to which you fall heir, the one you most frequently have to fight off for yourself is the common cold. You have probably resigned yourself to these miseries in the past. "Nothing really helps," people have told you. "A cold lasts a week if you dose yourself up, and seven days if you don't."

The picture need not be that grim. Look at these practical, effective measures, which you can take right in your own home.

SPEED COLD RECOVERY WITH SIMPLE MEANS

Shorten colds with better drainage. Your body has a very effective way of fighting off any germs that try to gain a foothold within its tissues. Thousands of germ-devouring white blood cells get to the scene in a matter of moments. Each of these cells stuffs itself with germs. As long as there is some place for the stuffed, useless white blood cells to go, your body washes them away on a wave of fluid and sends other germ-devouring white blood cells in their place.

That's why good drainage helps your nose and sinuses. A cold makes your nose lining swell and closes off pockets of infection. If you shrink your swollen nose lining with proper drops, trapped pus can drain away. A new horde of white blood cells can get to work, throwing off your infection.

Nose drops help shorten colds and make sinus infection less likely. When your nose is clogged, pockets of infection in the nasal cavity and in the sinuses cannot drain properly. You need nose drops as soon as the stuffed-up stage of a cold develops, or whenever you get sinus discomfort. There are at least two effective preparations which you can get from your druggist without prescription. Either of these will open up a stuffy nose and make you feel better, as well as giving better drainage:

> Neosynephrine Hydrochloride ¼ % in Isotonic Saline
> Ephedrine 1 % in Isotonic Saline

You can use nose drops in perfect safety if you follow a few simple rules:

> See your doctor before using nose drops if you have severe high blood pressure or heart disease. Blood vessel shrinking ingredients raise your blood pressure and speed heart action somewhat, which may aggravate these disorders.
>
> Use the drops every three hours if necessary for two or three days at the height of a cold, but quit by the end of a week to avoid rebound congestion. After prolonged use, allergy to these compounds usually makes your nose lining swell an hour or so after you use them. When you use more drops to combat the resulting stuffiness, you get into a vicious circle that sometimes lasts for months or years.
>
> Use only two or three drops of neosynephrine or ephedrine in each nostril at a time. If this much doesn't work, wait 10 minutes and repeat once. The first dose should shrink the reachable nose lining so that the second dose can get at still-swollen areas for complete relief.

How to use nose drops. You can get much more help from nose drops if they soak into the part of your nose lining where the sinus openings and hidden pockets of infection are located. Squirt straight up the nose passage toward the center of your forehead with an atomizer. Or use this special position so that the nose drops puddle around the sinus openings:

> Lie on your back with two pillows under your shoulder blades or with your head hanging over the side of the bed. Be sure that your head is lower than your shoulders. Now turn your chin to your right, so that it points toward your right shoulder. Put drops into your right nostril. Wait 30 seconds. Turn your head toward the left, and put drops into your left nostril. After 30 seconds, sit up and lean your head forward for a few seconds.

Tiny time pills. Contac, Ornade and several other cold capsules contain an ingredient which shrinks the blood vessels in your nose lining. This gives relief similar to that from nose drops without the danger of rebound congestion. Most patients would rather swallow a capsule every twelve hours than use drops every three or four, so I've been giving capsules as first choice in people with totally normal blood pressure and circulation. Side effects usually include temporary boost in blood pressure, somewhat faster pulse, and sometimes an overstimulated, drawn-tight type of nervousness. If these effects might add to an existing problem, it's better to stick with drops.

Soothing spray or snuffling solution. After the first three to seven days of a cold, most nasal stuffiness and sinus blockage is usually due to thick mucus instead of swollen nose lining. At this point you should stop using neosynephrine or ephedrine drops. However, you usually can get a great deal of relief by thinning the thick material. Easy techniques: Either spray or snuff up a soothing, mucus-thinning solution into your nose. Use this recipe:

> 1 level teaspoonful table salt.
> 1 pint distilled water.
> 2—4 drops Eau de Cologne if desired for pleasant scent.

If you do not have distilled water, you can use tap water by letting it stand overnight in a shallow pan to allow the chlorine to escape. Use with an atomizer, or pour a couple of teaspoonfuls into the hollow of your hand and snuff it up. One such spraying or snuffing every three to four hours usually keeps the passages open.

Get better more quickly, more safely, and more cheaply by holding antibiotics in reserve. Penicillin works wonders against germs it can attack. It is absolutely worthless for anything caused by a virus, particularly colds, flu, and ordinary sore throats. Four out of five doses of penicillin given for colds or sore throats are actually worthless or harmful. If you hold penicillin and other germ killers in reserve, you will avoid many serious drug allergies. You will get more effective care for complications like ear or sinus infections, which are just as frequent and much more stubborn when penicillin is used for the original cold. And you will save money.

How can you hold penicillin in reserve? Don't take penicillin on your own, either by buying a supply without a doctor's prescription or by starting on left-over medicine from a previous illness. Take care of milder colds and sore throats for yourself, with the measures described in this chapter. If a severe cold drives you to your doctor, tell him that you'll be especially pleased if he can get you through without using germ killers. And don't go to a doctor who prescribes germ killers without a careful examination and a blood count. A doctor who decides that you need penicillin after one look at your nose and throat isn't giving you scientific treatment: he's playing a lazy man's guessing game.

Make colds briefer, avoid sinus trouble, and keep your hearing sharper by controlled nose blowing. Want to cut your colds to only three days each, even if they've been averaging two weeks or longer? That's what a young Air Force doctor did for his charges during World War II. The main feature of his cold program didn't require any complicated steps: it was to cut down nose blowing.

Your nose is always loaded with dangerous germs. Some of the spaces with which it is linked, like the sinuses and the cavities of the ears, normally have no germs in them at all. Sweeper cells guard the entrances to these spaces, but sweep only at a very slow rate. They can't keep ahead of a burst of air pushed by a cough or a sneeze. They can't keep ahead of the blast you make whenever you blow your nose.

That's why you can cut the length of your colds, cut your chance of getting sinus trouble, and decrease the biggest single danger to your sharp hearing by taking a single step: throw away your handkerchief and try to forget nose-blowing!

The habit of a lifetime is hard to break. Sniff and swallow. Wipe your nose gently. But if you find yourself blowing before you know it, blow gently with both nostrils open. Never stop up the free nostril to blast open the closed-over one. Settle for one breathing space if you must, but don't blast yourself into a miserable sinus infection.

Rest to build up your resistance. The fastest way to beat a cold is undoubtedly in bed. Second best is a day broken with rest intervals: at least one half-hour rest at lunch time or before supper, plus ten hours in bed at night.

Aspirin. If aches and pains disturb your rest, take two aspirin tablets after each meal and at bedtime whether you feel as if you need them or not. Take aspirin by the day, not by the ache: on and off dosage sometimes kicks your fever curve up and down, making for extra sweats and chilly sensations. This amount of aspirin is perfectly safe. The after-meals timing almost always prevents nausea. Take aspirin regularly throughout the cold, until aches and pains have thoroughly subsided.

Some people, particularly children, get better effect by alternating aspirin with aminopyrine (Datril), also available without prescription in most states. In this way you can get the same relief from aches and pains and fever with half as much of each medicine. Follow the same four times a day schedule, but take aspirin one time and Datril the next.

Dodge he-man germs during a cold. One person in five who starts with an ordinary cold or sore throat gets some further infection before he gets well. A cold weakens your body's defenses so that you get sick from germs which you could ordinarily fight off with ease. But here's a hopeful fact: the germs that cause serious infections are seldom in your nose or throat when the original cold strikes. *If you can dodge new germ families for the first few days of a cold, you can cut your chance of sinus or chest infection at least in half.*

Children's Dosages

You can calculate the proper dosage for most medicines, including aspirin and cough preparations, by following the table devised at Guy's Hospital, London. To use this table, first determine the safe adult dose from package literature or label. BE VERY CAREFUL TO DISTINGUISH "GRAINS" (ABBREVIATED GR.) FROM "GRAMS" (ABBREVIATED GM.) WHICH ARE FIFTEEN TIMES AS LARGE. Determine the content of a child's size tablet or the strength of a teaspoonful (one dram or 5 cc) of liquid, and figure from there.

Age	Fraction of Adult Dose	Age	Fraction of Adult Dose
1 month	1/20	3 years	1/5
3 months	1/15	4 years	1/4
6 months	1/10	5 & 6 years	1/3
9 months	1/9	7 & 8 years	1/2
1 year	1/7	10 & 12 years	2/3
2 years	1/6	13 & 15 years	3/4

How can you dodge new germ families? Fortunately, most of them actually come from other members of your family or circle of friends. You can cut your germ exposure tremendously by taking three simple steps:

1. Avoid germ-laden mouth moisture. Sanitation will never make mankind give up the kiss. But why not refrain during colds, and shift to the cheek when in doubt? Why share one bathroom glass with the whole household? Small plastic glasses cost only a few cents apiece. One for each member of your family, perhaps colored to match his toothbrush, will take up very little space. Likewise with mouth-touching toys, food from other people's plates and so on.

2. Spray-rinse dishes and let them drain dry. The best germ-dodging policy actually saves work here! Dishes are much more free of germs if they are sprayed or rinsed with very hot water and left to dry than if you work them over with a towel.

3. Use space to prevent germ spread. Most of the germs which people spread into the air when they talk are in relatively large droplets. These fall to the ground within six feet. Chairs arranged so the people's heads are six feet apart let many less germs pass from person to person in your living room, dinning room, and office or shop.

These three steps—avoiding mouth moisture, spray-rinsing dishes, and keeping at moderate distance—keep down the number of excess germs you face while a cold is cutting down your body's power to fight.

HOW TO FIGHT COLD-PRONENESS

Almost anyone can substantially reduce his exposure to cold germs and substantially increase his resistance to them. If you are particularly subject to colds, home measures to counteract this tendency usually prove especially worthwhile. These measures are more effective than any cold shot yet devised, and involve absolutely no medical expense or risk.

You cannot dodge cold germs simply by avoiding people who sneeze and cough. Colds spread mainly before complaints begin, and reach you mainly from members of your own family or close circle of friends. A few germs, even of the worst possible kind, do you no harm. It takes thousands or millions of germs, all from the same germ family, to set up disease. Even one less than the crucial number leads to no trouble at all. You can cut down spread of germs through mouth moisture, improperly sanitized dishes, and close quarters in the firm knowledge that even a few less germs spread may mean a great deal less sickness in your household.

Protect your nose lining against cold germs. Some home measures for preventing colds are just common sense: enough rest, well-chosen foods, and sufficient warm clothing. Science can add two tremendous aids: extra help for your body's main shield against cold germs, which is your nose lining, and heightened resistance through cold-fighting morale.

How your nose lining protects you against germs. Your nose lining spreads an invisibly thin sheet of sticky mucus over the entire inside of your nose. When you breathe in germs, most of them stick in the sheet of mucus. Tiny sweeper cells continually brush the mucus back into your throat. A brand new sheet forms every six minutes or so. Meanwhile sweepings pile up at the back of your throat until they make a glob big enough for you to swallow. Your stomach acids kill the germs.

In the wintertime, the dry, heated air turns your nose lining's mucus blanket to crusts. It may even dry the nose lining until it cracks, providing completely free access to germs. Moisturization prevents this effect, and thus increases your nose lining's resistance.

How can you moisturize your nose lining? Three main methods are worthwhile:

1. Add moisture to heated air. Humidifiers or moisturizing pans on the radiators are worthwhile. They at least take the edge off the dryness of indoor air. They cannot do the whole job, since thorough home air moisturization requires evaporation of several gallons of water each day.

2. Turn down the heat. When you warm air from 68 degrees to 80 degrees, you increase its drying power more than fourfold. It's best to heat your house only to 68 degrees and put on extra sweaters or heavier clothes for bodily warmth. At night, you can cool your bedroom five or ten degrees by turning heat down or by ventilation. That gives your nose lining a rest from too-dry, overheated air. Extra blankets keep your body comfortably warm.

3. Use home-made moisturizing nose spray. You can banish dry crusts and help your nose's defense by using this moisturizing spray:

> 1 tablespoonful glycerin, obtained from any drugstore
>   without prescription.
> 1½ tablespoonfuls 70% alcohol (rubbing alcohol strength).
> 1 teaspoonful table salt.
> 1 pint tap or distilled water.

If your tap water has a heavy odor of chlorine, let it stand overnight in an open vessel. Mix the ingredients and stir until salt is thoroughly dissolved. Pour into clean bottle and stopper firmly.

Get a plastic pocket atomizer for about 50¢ at the drugstore, fill it with this solution, and use it several times a day as needed.

Last-minute action to ward off a cold. Can you tell when a cold is just coming on? If you can, you may be able to stop some colds from getting a real start.

The first thing to try is moisturizing spray (see above). Spray the inside of your nose thoroughly every hour or two. Keep warm and get a good night's sleep. This program alone will stop some colds in their tracks.

If you have enough colds to make it worthwhile, one other medicine might help you. It's a combination of codeine and papaverine, which are available on prescription only. When used at the first sign of a cold, it sometimes stops the nose lining responses which allow germs to get a foothold. When you next see your doctor, ask him if you should have this material on hand and how you should use it when you feel a cold coming on.

Vitamin C keeps cropping up as a cold-fighting aid. Years ago, it was very popular in 25-50 mgm doses "at the first sign of a cold." Studies with similar-looking sugar pills showed no real effect from this dosage. Under its new name of "ascorbic acid" Vitamin C has recently been advised in doses of 250-500 mgms "when you first feel a cold coming on." Some world-recognized experts have given this dosage their support, but I haven't seen any definite proof. Trouble is that everyone thinks he's going to get a cold several times as often as he actually gets one, so studies done without the sugar pill routine are subject to error. Vitamin C won't hurt you, though, if you want to give it a try.

Fight colds by mental measures. Parts of your brain actually govern your circulation and many other bodily functions through which you fight off germs. Your emotional state greatly influences these functions. It can thus help or hurt your resistance to all kinds of infection. This effect is very strong. Just thinking you are liable to get a cold may tip the balance and make you fall victim to one.

A research expert proved the importance of emotions to the origin of colds without even trying. He wanted to grow cold germs in the laboratory. In order to tell whether the germs were present in his culture solution, he decided to spray some into a few people's noses. The subjects were kept in hospital rooms and protected from new infections until any strong germs they already had acquired would have shown up. (Some cold germs are probably present in most people's throats all the time, but not enough to cause a cold so long as their resistance is normal.) Then he sprayed a few people with ordinary water, telling them the stuff was loaded with germs. One out of five promptly came down with a cold.

The rest of the experiment proved that strong cold germs were present in the doctor's other mixture. But this very first step proved a point which is very important to you. It means that even weak cold germs can be helped along by mental forces until they overcome your resistance. When you get chilled or feel a draught, the chances are that you say to yourself: "Now I'm in for it! I'll have a cold tomorrow for sure!" That conviction itself causes concern and emotional response which actually help to give you the cold.

Build your cold fighting morale. You can protect yourself against two thirds of all colds by building cold-fighting morale. That's what a team of researchers at Michigan found out when they were experimenting with a new cold vaccine. They thought they had an effective product, and designed tests to prove the fact. One group of people got the vaccine. Another group got nothing, and still another got distilled water, being told that they were getting cold shots.

When the results were in, the people who took the cold shots reported only one third as many colds as the ones who had nothing at all. But the ones who got the distilled water had even less! The conviction that they would get less colds actually cut the number of colds these people suffered tremendously!

What does this mean to you? Certainly not that your colds aren't real: they're real, germ-caused infections. But your resistance may be affected so much by concern about old wives' tales that you have many colds which you would otherwise fight off.

This need not be. You can use mental forces to *increase* your resistance instead of impair it. You can build your cold-fighting morale to the point where you have many less colds per year.

How to build cold-fighting morale. Cold-fighting morale is best built on one firm conviction: *nothing that happens to you can give you a cold.* You need never say to yourself: "Drat it! I did thus-and-so, so now I'll probably get a cold!" Absolutely none of the common experiences you might note can give you a cold.

Let's look at some of the ideas science has explored in reaching this conclusion:

Draughts, night air, and going without a hat do not cause colds. The lining of your nose is definitely affected by nerve and emotional balance. Your nose can get stopped up or runny on the basis of pure nerve reflex when you are exposed to wind or cold. It can get stopped up and runny after any uncomfortable nerve-tickling exposure, even through slight draughts. But unless worry or concern add further burdens, your nose lining will usually get back to normal before the ever-present cold germs actually get a start.

Chilling doesn't cause colds. When I was only a child, I remember my aunt stomping her feet one day as she came in the front door.

"Brrrr—" she said. "I'm chilled clean through. Have a cold tomorrow, like as not."

The next day, sure enough! She had a cold. But today's science says that my aunt probably already had the cold germs in her body, and those germs were already starting disease when she first walked in my door and said "Brrrr—." My aunt almost certainly felt chilly because of a beginning cold; she didn't get the cold because of the chill. But millions of people are positive that whenever they get chilled a cold will certainly follow. If they actually do get chilled, not simply get chilly sensations because of a beginning cold, how many of them actually suffer a cold, not because of the chill, but because of fearful certainty that they are headed for the sickbed?

Have confidence in your body's powers. Of course, it pays to dress yourself warmly and to avoid extreme exposure. But it pays to have confidence in your body, too. Take reasonable measures to avoid chilling, then shrug your shoulders and forget it if you find that you've been uncomfortably cool.

Other people's colds aren't easy to catch. Suppose a stranger sneezes at you in a store. What are your chances of getting a cold?

Actually, almost none at all. Children, who take little care to dodge other people's germs, get colds four times out of five when they are right in the household with a cold victim. But as an adult, you will *escape* four times out of five even if you are in close family contact with a cold. Moreover, most people who sneeze or cough at you in public have already passed the early days when their cold can still be spread, and could not give you germs no matter how hard they tried. Many people sneeze or cough because of conditions which are impossible to spread, like allergy. Your chance of catching a stranger's cold is almost zero, but your chance of worrying yourself into a cold after he's sneezed in your face is considerable indeed, unless you can become convinced that colds rarely spread through such contact.

Cold-fighting morale can really protect you. If you are convinced that nothing is likely to cause colds, you won't suffer psychologically induced ones. You will probably also increase your resistance against whatever cold-causing germs you meet. So whenever you find yourself thinking that what has just happened might cause a cold, repeat to yourself several times: "Nothing that happens to me can give me a cold. Not draughts, not chilling, not even a victim's sneeze! Nothing that happens to me can give me a cold!" As you go about your daily activities, have confidence in your body's powers of resistance. You will still occasionally meet an overwhelming number of cold germs and suffer an infection. But you can throw off the bulk of cold germs without even a sniffle.

ORDINARY SORE THROAT, LARYNGITIS, AND COUGH

More and more mild infections of the upper breathing passages seem to be showing up as sore or scratchy throats instead of ordinary colds. Most victims complain of soreness with slight fever or chilly sensations, headache, and muscular discomfort. After 12 to 24 hours, the trouble spreads both up and down: stuffiness in the back of the nose with some thick mucus usually starts first, then soreness beneath the upper part of the breastbone. A dry, uncomfortable cough is often troublesome, especially at night. The severe complaints usually settle down in about a week, but your throat may feel scratchy and an ordinary day's work may prove unusually fatiguing for two or three weeks.

Most of the measures you would use for a common cold prove helpful here: rest, germ shunning, aspirin, and nose drops and sprays as needed. These further measures give additional relief:

Hot gargles. What is the best solution to use as a mouthwash or gargle? One of my doctor friends settled this question by actually using different preparations, then determining how many germs were left. His surprising conclusion: ordinary salt water works just as well as any antiseptics tested. Reason: all the germs on the surface where antiseptics can reach them wash away promptly anyway. Germs down the sewer do you no more harm alive than dead.

Frequent gargling removes germs. One-half teaspoonful of table salt to a glassful of water is as effective as any gargling solution you can buy. You can add considerably to the soothing effect of gargles by making them quite hot: as hot as you can stand without burning. Hot salt water gargles four times a day help to keep you comfortable and speed your recovery.

Hot irrigations. The rawness of a virus sore throat often extends so far back that gargling just doesn't seem to reach it. In this case, or if you have difficulty gargling effectively, the best home measure is the hot irrigation. Fit the glass tip from an ordinary eyedropper to the end of a household enema apparatus (fountain syringe). Make an irrigating solution by adding four level teaspoonfuls of table salt to two quarts of very warm water, as hot as you can use comfortably without burning (112° F.). Arrange the enema bag 24 inches above the level at which you will irrigate. Lean over a washbasin with your head tipped forward and your mouth open. Squirt the water back into your throat, directing the stream toward the sore area. You won't choke and you need not spit: the water will run back out into the basin. Pause occasionally to breathe. If gagging occurs, direct the stream a bit lower—the problem is usually that the solution has forced the uvula back against the sensitive back wall of your pharynx. Repeat until all the solution is used up.

You can use throat irrigations several times a day for ordinary sore throat. Smoldering throat problems which cause soreness mainly in the morning yield especially well to this measure.

Throat-soothing syrups. An ordinary sore throat soon settles down to the stage of morning rawness and dry, harsh feeling, which yields very well to loosening-type cough syrups. Syrup of cocillana, available at your drugstore in such preparations as Syrup of Cosanyl, works especially well. Cough mixtures containing ipecac and ammonium chloride such as Lilly's Mentholated Expectorant are also effective.

Laryngitis. Virus sore throats sometimes settle in the voice box, causing hoarseness or complete loss of voice and a brassy, tight-feeling cough. In severe cases, or if breathing becomes difficult, you need your doctor's help. The much commoner, mild form of laryngitis often yields to these home measures:

Steam. You can usually get a great deal of relief and definitely speed healing of laryngitis by breathing moist, steamy air for at least a half an hour three or four times a day. Make a steam tent on your bed by opening an umbrella, laying it on its side with the top toward the head of the bed, and covering it with a sheet. Put a hot plate on the floor beside the bed, and start a kettle of water boiling on it. Use the core from a roll of paper towels or a rolled piece of heavy wrapping paper held together with several rubber bands to lead the steam up into your tent. Steam gives great help for croup and childhood coughs, many of which are forms of laryngitis. The safety problems of such care make it almost too dangerous to use, though. Youngsters become restless and unreliable when ill. Anything hot in their vicinity becomes a great hazard, either through scalding or through shifting of the sheets or bedclothing into the source of heat. Fortunately, there is a way to eat your cake and have it, too—"cold steamers," which actually work by throwing out a mist of very fine water droplets instead of boiling the water into steam, give just about the same benefits without burn risk. Any drugstore can supply such a unit for about $10—substantial expense, but cheap as insurance against a painful and disabling burn.

Voice rest. A husky voice means that your vocal cords are swollen, red and raw. If any surface part of your body—say your finger—were swollen, red, and raw, you would carefully spare it from any unnecessary use. Why not do the same thing with your voice? Most patients find that if they can absolutely stop talking for two days, carrying a notebook and pencil with which to write notes for essential communications, they usually get well. If this is impossible for you, spare your voice as much as you can.

Cough looseners. You can control laryngitic cough fast by taking simultaneously:

1 teaspoonful paregoric.
1 teaspoonful castor oil.
1 teaspoonful syrup of ipecac.

All of these preparations are available at your drugstore without prescription. The paregoric cancels out the laxative action of the castor oil, but leaves its very potent action on glands in the breathing passages unimpaired. If you cannot get any syrup of ipecac promptly, syrup of cosillana or most other common cough-loosening syrups will do. A dose of this triple-threat cough remedy every four hours relieves the tightness and cough of laryngitis quite well.

Warmth. Laryngitis is very sensitive to temperature change. You will get well much more quickly if you stay at home with hoarseness. If you must go out, wear a double muffler or wool scarf around your neck.

Dilute nitric acid. If prompt restoration of your voice is absolutely essential, you may find treatment with dilute nitric acid worthwhile. Among others, I have prescribed this method for three different ministers who were still voiceless by Saturday night. Each was ready for the pulpit by Sunday morning. The method is absolutely safe if you follow three precautions:

1. Be sure you get *dilute* nitric acid, whose strength is designated 0.1 Normal. Full strength or chemically pure nitric acid is designated 12 Normal, and is 120 times too strong.

2. Add ten drops of dilute nitric acid to half a glass of water for each treatment. *Do not use it straight from the bottle.*

3. Sip the diluted mixture through a glass straw held well inside your mouth to avoid the slight speeding of cavity formation which might result from contact of the acid with your teeth.

Three or four doses at two hour intervals restore the voice in most cases.

Home measures for cough. You can decide which coughs will probably yield quickly to home measures and which need medical attention right away. Your doctor can give worthwhile help if:

1. Your temperature goes over 100 degrees.

2. You get severe headache, aches and pains, and chilly sensations.

3. You spit up bloodstreaked or rusty-looking phlegm.

4. Your appetite is off, so that you are losing weight.

5. The cough is accompanied by pain in the chest, other than a tight feeling under the upper part of the breastbone, by pain on breathing deeply, or by shortness of breath.

6. The cough produces more than two tablespoons of pus-filled or foul-smelling phlegm before breakfast time.

7. The cough fails to respond promptly to home measures.

Tight coughs. When the rawness from a cold or ordinary sore throat spreads down into your windpipe, you get a tight, dry cough. You do not spit up much phlegm or feel it rattling around in your chest as you do with a loose cough. A tearing sensation may clutch at your chest with each paroxysm. Cough may be especially annoying when you first lie down at night, and shortly after any spurt of activity or exertion.

Benzoin and steam. Steam inhalation helps this kind of cough a great deal. A teaspoonful of compound tincture of benzoin makes the steam even more soothing. Benzoin stains the inside of the pan: unless you have an old kettle you want to use for steaming only, it's best to float a shallow tin can or a tray-shaped piece of heavy aluminum foil inside the kettle and put the benzoin inside *that*. Many patients find that steaming for an hour or more four times a day is very worthwhile, although shorter periods also help. If you use this treatment for children, stay with them constantly. Read a story for them to keep down restlessness, and don't turn your back for an instant—the burn hazard from any steam source hot enough to vaporize the benzoin is very real indeed.

Cough syrups. Almost all of the nonprescription cough syrups are cough-loosening agents, and many of them work very well. If you haven't been satisfied with the product you have in your medicine chest now, try taking two teaspoonfuls of syrup of cosillana every three hours. Brown mixture is another excellent and inexpensive cough mixture.

Aspirin. A severe cough often causes enough discomfort to call for relief. Try aspirin first, two tablets if you weigh 150 pounds or less, three if you weigh more.

Many cough syrups include codeine or opium, which reinforce aspirin's pain relief. For children, scale down doses according to the table on page 102.

Patients with tight cough usually ask about chest rubs, greases, counterirritants, and plasters. These may give some relief, but in my experience not enough to make the disturbed rest and discomfort they involve worthwhile. Soaking the feet in very hot water also has some reflex cough-loosening action, but the water must be so hot that patients often burn themselves. For these reasons, I usually advise against these methods.

Loose cough. Mild varieties of loose cough usually are due to mucus and irritants that ooze down from the back of the nasal passages into the throat, windpipe, and bronchial tubes. You can attack this type of cough in several simple ways:

Salt water snuffling. If you keep the material which sweeps back into your throat thin enough, you can swallow it down without a single cough. Simplest technique: mix half a level teaspoonful of table salt in a glass of lukewarm water, pour a tablespoonful or so into the cupped palm of your hand, and snuffle it up into the nose. Repeat until the passages are clear of thick or irritating clots of mucus. Salt water can also be used in an atomizer if one is available.

Better drainage through controlled sleep posture. When you lie on your back, mucus and irritants from your nose run back into your throat and down your windpipe continually. On your side, this action is almost as great. But when you lie face down, your breathing passages drain outward from the bottom of your windpipe to the tip of your nose. Most patients are not comfortable flat on their abdomens when they have a cough, so I usually recommend putting one pillow underneath the right side of the chest and bending the right knee slightly to keep the body about one-quarter rolled toward the left.

Special gravity-aided lung drainage. If you get a deep, loose type cough, you may have a lot of trouble raising all the phlegm that accumulates in your chest. First thing in the morning, and several times throughout the day as moisture begins to accumulate, you should try this program:

> Lie face down across your bed with a footstool or sturdy wooden box at the bedside just beneath your head. Slide forward until only your hips and legs remain on the bed, with your head and chest dangling almost straight downward. Prop your elbows on the stool or box to achieve reasonable comfort, and take several deep breaths or coughs. Remain in this position for about ten minutes, taking a few deep breaths or coughs every two minutes or so. Do not attempt to swallow phlegm that you raise while in this position: keep a basin or a supply of tissues in reach so that you can spit it out.

Cough syrups and remedies. If bursts of coughing disturb your rest or interfere greatly with jobs you simply must do, you need effective cough controlling medicine. Your druggist can sell without prescription several ready-mixed preparations containing completely safe amounts of codeine or other cough-suppressing opium elements such as elixir of terpin hydrate with codeine, or brown mixture with opium. With severe night cough, you may find standard strength cough mixtures do not give enough relief. One way to control cough without taking an overdose is to supplement cough syrup with paregoric, which contains cough suppressing opium without other cough syrup ingredients. A teaspoonful of brown mixture with opium plus a teaspoonful of paregoric brings your total dosage very close to that supplied by strong prescription cough preparations. Like any powerful cough-suppressing combination, this occasionally causes nausea or constipation in sensitive people. If your cough robs you of too much sleep, though, the results you will get with this mixture may well be worth the slight risk of digestive upset.

Rest. Mild type coughs are still infections, even though they seldom involve germs of a kind your doctor could kill with penicillin. You can definitely build your recuperative powers with rest. Half an hour in bed before supper and ten hours of rest at night is my usual recommendation.

Fluids. The classic advice is to drink lots of juice, water, and pop. Cola beverages, coffee, and tea should not be used beyond the amounts to which you are accustomed, because they contain enough stimulant to cause restlessness or gas cramps when used in large quantity. Ginger ale, fruit flavored pop, and mixtures of fruit juice and ginger ale often sit especially well. Probably the main benefit you get from this program is control of the bowel problems which otherwise often follow upon decreased activity, fever, poor appetite, and constipating medications. I don't advise alcoholic beverages as a means of forcing fluids, since alcohol combines with a great deal of water in the process of burning inside your body (as everyone who has suffered morning-after thirst can tell).

CHAPTER EIGHT

How to Control Dragged-out and Recurring Miseries of the Nose, Throat, and Sinuses

Many dragged-out or recurring nose, throat, and sinus miseries cause considerable suffering without quite driving you to your doctor's office. You've more or less learned to live with your smoldering sinus discomfort. Each individual attack of hay fever is half over before you can find time for a doctor visit. So you bear up as best you can.

You'll find that proper home measures make these disorders much easier to bear. You can probably get considerable relief from sore or crusted nose, sinus trouble, and chronic sore throat with simple home measures. Drainage back into your throat with constant tickle or "smoker's cough" may yield entirely to home measures. You may rid yourself entirely of nosebleeds, stuffy nose, hay or rose fever, allergic rhinitis and even asthma with home measures. The rugged Minnesota climate gives us plenty of chance to try different home measures against these ailments. Here are the remedies my patients have found most effective.

NASAL CRUSTING, SORE NOSE, AND NOSEBLEEDS

Some of the commonest and most easily corrected nasal miseries stem from the irritating dryness of the air you breathe. The more you heat air, the drier it becomes, which makes the indoor air positively crackle during Minnesota winters. Even in areas with milder weather, nasal crusts or boogies form just inside the nose, causing considerable discomfort and stuffiness. You almost can't help picking at these crusts at times, causing soreness, nosebleeds. and infection. Dry air often causes nosebleeds, too: the spot where most nosebleeds start is just inside the nose on the wall between the two nostrils, where the nose lining is stretched thin and easily dried to the cracking point.

Nasal crusts. You can probably save yourself a great deal of nagging discomfort by controlling nasal crusts. Moisturizing measures (used for cold prevention, as explained above) may also control crusts. If not, try these techniques:

Nose lining anointment. You can usually prevent all crusting, most nose soreness, and a substantial share of nosebleeds by anointing your nose lining with lanolin or petroleum jelly. Most of my patients use this measure about three times a week during the heating season, and perhaps once a week during warm weather. More frequent self-treatment is perfectly safe if it proves desirable. Here are detailed directions:

> Obtain one ounce of lanolin from your druggist. Dip up a glob slightly larger than a match head with the tip of your right index finger or with a cotton-tipped applicator. Gently press the tip of your nose straight upward with the tip of your left index finger, and apply the lanolin to the front corner of the wall between the nostrils about a quarter-inch up from the opening. As the lanolin melts, it will spread over the entire nose lining layer.
>
> If lanolin is not readily available or if you find its smell objectionable, use *unmedicated* white petroleum jelly. Probably you will need two or three times as many applications of petroleum jelly as of lanolin, but it does just as good a job.
>
> CAUTION: NEITHER LANOLIN NOR PETROLEUM JELLY SHOULD BE USED BELOW AGE TWELVE. Underdeveloped childhood "sweeper" cells cannot handle oily substances, and allow them to trickle down into the lungs, occasionally causing serious disease.

Tap water snuffling. If nasal crusts or dryness already plague you, the temptation to pick or blow at them is almost intolerable. Any measure which softens the crusts will let your nose lining's sweeper cells carry them away. If you sniff up a teaspoonful or two of warm tap water from the palm of your hand, you can usually restore nasal comfort without harmful picking or blowing. The high chlorine content makes most tap water slightly more harsh than moisturizing spray, but not harmfully so. The amount of water you can hold on your palm will not fill the cavern of your nose and will not cause gagging or get into your windpipe.

Sore nose. A red, sore swelling of the side of the nose just above the nostril frequently results from pull on the hair roots inside the nose, either by crusts or while clipping protruding nasal hair. If you suffer from this condition, *do not pick or squeeze the sore area.* The veins which carry blood away from this spot lead back through the brain cage in many people. Squeezing or picking can occasionally result in very serious spread of infection along those veins. You can never be sure whether you have the dangerous variety of circulation until too late, so it's best to take no chance of stirring up a brain abscess or other deadly disorder. Instead, use heat to draw out or heal the infection. Apply wet cloths which are as hot as is comfortable without burning (112 degrees), cover with a dry towel to help hold the heat, and change every five minutes or so to keep the temperature right. Each application should last at least half an hour. Every two hours is about the right frequency. If soreness spreads, chills and fever develop, or the tissue around the eye begins to swell, call your doctor.

Nosebleeds. If you have a nosebleed, nine times out of ten it originates in the wall between your nostrils just behind the tip of your nose. To control a nosebleed, try these five steps:

Patience and proper position. By sitting up in a quiet and relaxed position, you cut down the pressure in the nasal blood vessels. This often helps normal processes of repair. Ordinarily, your head should be tipped slightly forward so that the blood runs out of your nose instead of back into your throat. Otherwise, swallowed blood often irritates the stomach, adding nausea and vomiting to your other problems. If you become dizzy or faint in the upright position, you may need to lie down temporarily: if so, lie partly on your face and partly on your side with pillows to support you.

Cold compresses. A cold cloth on the bridge of the nose or forehead sometimes seems to contract the bleeding vessels and help stop them up.

Nasal packs. A half-inch-wide strip of facial tissue or a wisp of cotton helps to give flowing blood a matrix on which to clot. Double the pack over the blunt end of a pencil and insert it gently straight up toward the forehead, about three-quarters of an inch. Touch the pack against the wall between your nostrils, and twist the pencil slightly to disengage it. Withdraw the pencil, leaving the pack in place. Pick up another fold of the pack material two or three inches down and follow the same procedure until the nasal passage is full. No great pressure is required.

Pressure between fingers. If the bleeding continues in spite of the pack, gently press the sides of your nose together between your thumb and forefinger, increasing pressure on the pack. Continue the pressure for at least five minutes by the clock before releasing it to see whether bleeding still continues.

Clothespin pressure. Some patients seem to get better results by using a pincer-type clothespin with a couple of layers of handkerchief for padding, which they leave in place for 10 to 15 minutes.

Removing the pack. If a nasal pack or a pack plus pressure finally stops a nosebleed, you should leave the pack in place for 3 to 12 hours. Otherwise, the bleeding often starts again when you remove the pack. If you have used cotton, you can moisten it with mild salt water (one-half teaspoon to a glassful of water) several times over a five minute period before attempting to remove it. Packing can be replaced if fresh bleeding starts, but should not be left in place for over 24 hours. See your doctor if bleeding continues after that interval.

Follow-up treatment. In most cases, the lanolin program described above prevents further nosebleeds. However, nosebleeds sometimes are due to high blood pressure, disease of the blood, or rheumatic fever, for which medical treatment is very worthwhile. Frequent or severe nosebleeds, or nosebleeds accompanied by other complaints such as headache, joint pains, or fever, certainly deserve your doctor's care.

HOME CARE FOR SINUS MISERIES, STUFFY NOSE, CHRONIC SORE THROAT, AND POSTNASAL DRIP

Sinus blockage or irritation causes pain. Infection which calls for prescription germ killers only occurs in about one-fifth of the cases. Among the patients with complaints severe enough and protracted enough to reach a specialist, a majority have infection. However, a British study based on *all* people with sinus complaints shows that four out of five have germ-free sinuses. My own experience almost exactly duplicates this figure. You can distinguish attacks that require your doctor's prompt attention by these signs:

1. Throbbing pain instead of steady, dull discomfort.
2. Fever.
3. Muscular aches and pains, loss of appetite and weakness.
4. Foul-smelling or opaque white or yellow matter draining back into the throat usually means infection. Translucent or semi-opaque mucus does not necessarily mean infection no matter what its color might be.

Home care when sinus pain strikes. Steady, bursting pain under the cheekbones or just above the eyes usually stems from sinus irritation. If you get such an attack, these measures may help:

Aspirin. Three aspirin tablets help to relieve the average 150 pounder. Adjust the dose up or down if your weight is 35 pounds or more from this standard.

Nose drops or spray. You can use the same nose drops or spray advised for colds (¼ per cent Neosynephrine or 1 per cent Ephedrine) for sinus miseries. However, these often prove somewhat weak, especially if you have had a great deal of previous trouble. One-half per cent Neosynephrine is safe for two or three applications to get the sinuses draining, and often proves worthwhile. Contac, Ornade or Neosynephrine tablets give similar but less localized effect.

Some sinus sufferers find that the position ordinarily advised for instilling nosedrops (see above) does not give very good effect. If this proves true, try lying on your right side with a pillow under your right shoulder and letting your head fall sideward so that your right ear is against your right shoulder. Put drops in the right side, wait half a minute, then switch position to do the left side.

Lightbulb baking. Many sinus sufferers find heat quite helpful. One convenient form is lightbulb baking. Place moist pledgets of cotton over your eyes. Place 100-watt bulbs in two lamps with metal reflectors, such as goosenecked desk lamps. If you have no lamps with metal reflectors, line the shades of ordinary lamps with aluminum foil. Place the lamps about three feet away from your face, and adjust them closer or farther away as necessary as the bulbs become hot and your face becomes accustomed to the warmth. At least 30 minutes of baking is usually best at a sitting. Treatment can be continued safely for several hours or repeated frequently throughout the day if necessary.

Hot applications. Wet heat sometimes works as well or better than baking. A folded towel dipped in hot water works very well. The water should be as hot as is comfortable without risk of burning (112°). A dry towel or piece of plastic sheeting such as a plastic refrigerator bag helps to cut evaporation and to hold the heat. Dip the towel as often as necessary to keep it hot for 20 to 30 minutes. Always test water temperature with the back of your hand or some part not being treated with heat: otherwise, you may become sufficiently accustomed to the warmth to burn yourself.

Nasal irrigation. To some extent, the thick mucus which has already passed into the nearby nasal cavity blocks drainage. You can remove this material without harmful nose blowing by gentle nasal irrigation. Use nose-drops or spray five to ten minutes before this treatment to open the nasal passages. Mix four teaspoonfuls of table salt with two quarts of warm water in an enema bag. Replace the enema tip with the glass portion of an eyedropper. Insert this part way into one nostril and compress the side of your nose gently with a fingertip to make it fit snugly. Lean your head slightly forward over a basin. Adjust the enema bag so that the water level in it is about 12 inches higher than your nose, and start the flow. Water should run into one nostril and out the other. If flow is sluggish, you may increase the pressure slightly by raising the bag or lowering your head, but *never* allow more than eighteen inches difference in height between the bag and your nose.

Nasal siphonage. If you have frequent or continual sinus misery, an additional refinement may be worthwhile. Attach another eye-dropper tip to a two-foot piece of rubber tubing. Put a little water in your washbasin and immerse this tube in such a way that water displaces all the air from inside. Clamp or pinch off the tube. Prepare for nasal irrigation as described in the last paragraph, fitting the irrigating tip into your right nostril. Fit the siphon tip into your left nostril leaving its free end under water in the basin. Don't let the tubing empty itself. Release both tubes simultaneously. The weight of the water in the downward-flowing siphon tube creates a suction which literally pulls matter out of the sinuses. If the siphonage is interrupted for any reason, refill the siphon tube with water to restore full action. After you have used about half the irrigating solution, clamp or pinch off both tubes again and reverse nostrils to complete the treatment.

How to control continual sinus discomfort, stuffy nose, chronic sore tnroat, and postnasal drip. If you have continual nose troubles, the chances are that irritation is at fault. If your doctor has never remarked about the wall between your nostrils being far out of line or about other defects of nasal structure, and if the signs of infection which we discussed a few pages back have not been present, these home measures may give considerable improvement:

Stop using medicated nose drops, sprays, and jellies. Agents which shrink the nasal lining frequently cause rebound congestion, actually causing considerable swelling after a brief interval of relief. Germ killing medicines and antihistamines often cause later rawness and swelling, too. I have seen patients who continued to suffer from a stuffy nose, postnasal drainage, and sinus pain over long periods—in one case, twelve miserable years—when discontinuing all nasal decongestants, germ killers, and antihistamines brought prompt relief. Long-continued nasal stuffiness often disappears completely or substantially improves if you cease using all such preparations for two weeks. You can make the uncomfortable trial period somewhat more bearable with moisturizing spray, swallowed decongestants (discussed below) and hot applications.

Home decongestant method. You can fight severe nasal congestion without irritating your nose lining by swallowing decongestant preparations instead of dropping them into your nose. Contac, Neosynephrine, Ornade and other "decongestant cold capsules" have such ingredients. A few patients get rebound nasal congestion from these preparations, too, but not as many as from drops. If you have any heart trouble, blood pressure elevation, or nervousness you should check with a doctor before using these preparations.

Moisturizing spray. You will probably find that soothing home-made moisturizing spray (formula on page 104) will help you with most smoldering nose and sinus miseries. In addition to its cold-fighting action, this preparation thins thick, mucoid matter which drains back into the throat in almost all forms of smoldering nasal trouble. Moisturizing spray lets you swallow draining material easily instead of having it hang through a dozen swallows or coughs. The thin glycerin film left by moisturizing spray helps to replace the normal moving mucus blanket which has often disappeared after long bouts of nasal trouble and medication. It startlingly helps many patients with a background of stuffiness and sinus misery through the years.

Restrain nose-blowing. Besides its infection-spreading effect, violent nose-blowing irritates the nasal lining and makes it become swollen and sensitive. Sometimes this leads to a vicious circle: more swelling and sensitivity causes stuffiness and annoyance, which makes you blow your nose, which causes still more swelling and sensitivity. Either don't blow, or if you must blow keep both nostrils open and blow gently. Perhaps salt or tap water snuffling will help get rid of secretions, too.

Use a chin binder if necessary. Morning sore throat often results when your mouth drops open during relaxed sleep, so that you breathe through your mouth instead of your nose. Try moisturization and lowered nighttime temparature. If these measures fail, tie a soft cloth around your chin from the top of your head to hold your mouth closed when you are completely relaxed.

Tunnel breathing and protective clothing. Your nasal lining may be quite sensitive to abrupt changes in temperature and humidity. Sometimes sinus membranes engorge themselves when cold air hits the overlying skin. If you are very subject to such difficulties, you need to protect your face and breathing passages from the cold.

Research aimed at helping people survive in the arctic wastes has produced one excellent answer to this problem: tunnel breathing. In the frozen North, this is done through a fur-lined tunnel which projects forward from a heavy hood. When you take a breath inside such a hood, most of the air you get is warm, moist air which you just breathed out into the hood and tunnel. Just enough fresh air enters to keep your body well supplied.

The hardy Minnesota lumbermen learned many years ago to accomplish the same goal with a properly arranged muffler or scarf. By winding a turn over an ordinary peaked cap, then bringing it loosely over the lower half of the face, they made a breathing tunnel that also served as a sheltered peep hole through which to view the snow covered wonders of our wintry world. If you use a scarf in this way, be sure to wind it so that you rebreathe warm air trapped in your peep hole tunnel instead of breathing through the material.

The plastic masks which many surgeons now use in place of the old gauze models have much the same effect. Air comes into your breathing passages only after having passed through a narrow, tortuous path across your warm cheek surfaces. The 3 M Company marketed "cold weather masks" of this type widely for a while, too. Although they didn't go over too well with the general public, some drugstores still have these in stock.

Waxen kernels. Smoldering infection in the throat or sinuses often shows up more through sore and swollen glands down the neck than through direct soreness. This is especially true of children, in whom waxen kernels may stand out like knots beneath the angles of the jaws. Use the same measures with waxen kernels you would apply to chronic sore throat or sinus, as above. These lymph glands are the filters with which your body catches germs as they try to invade your system. Clearing up the germ source gets rid of gland infection more readily than any treatment aimed at the glands themselves, and hot soaks or other measures may make the glands drain through the skin, leaving unsightly scars.

If lymph glands enlarge without clear-cut infection of the nose or throat or if enlargement persists, blood counts and other studies should be done. This means a doctor visit, of course.

Antihistamines. A stuffy nose often stems from allergy to dusts and pollens or from irritation by fumes, dry air, cold air or emotional upset. You can usually get relief from all of these types of congestion with antihistamine tablets or capsules, some of the best of which are now available without a prescription. Most of my stuffy nose patients need about four capsules a day. They usually take their medicine immediately after meals and at bedtime to avoid the slight indigestion which antihistamines sometimes cause when taken on an empty stomach. A few people get a little dopey or slow from antihistamines, so you should always take the first dose when you do not have to drive a car or operate dangerous machinery for a few hours.

Corrective measures against allergy. Smoldering nasal complaints of any sort may have an allergic background. Such origin is especially likely if:

Stuffiness and discharge are worse in the morning when you first get up. Even if sinus pain occurs later in the day, signs of nasal irritation first thing in the morning may mean that the whole problem is due to allergy.

Watery discharge, sneezing, and stuffiness follow tasks involving exposure to household dusts, visits to certain localities, or nearness to certain objects. Anything from Grandma's cat to mold in a moist basement may be responsible.

Complaints clear up during vacation trips or visits away from home, or vanish when you take antihistamines.

If your complaints might be related in any way to allergy, here are nine tried and true home remedies, which my patients have found helpful.

HOME MEASURES AGAINST ALLERGY

Minnesota's fabulous variety of trees and grasses, plus a profusion of weeds on its vast stretches of uncultivated land, make pollen allergy one of its commonest plagues. House dust, animal dander, and molds bother our hearty Swedes as much as other Americans, too. When one of my patients complains of frequent nose colds with no fever or muscular discomfort, I can be almost sure that he really has allergy instead of infection. Continual watery discharge, nasal stuffiness, and sneezing point toward allergic rhinitis, the perennial form of hay fever which allergy sufferers tend to develop either independently or as an aftermath of the pollen allergy season. Asthma and hay fever almost always stem from allergy to breathed-in substances, of course.

Home measures help tremendously in fighting these varieties of allergy-caused misery. As emergency aid when you suffer an attack, *antihistamine capsules or tablets* every four hours often bring relief. *Ephedrine,* either in capsule form or in half-teaspoonful swallowed doses of the standard one per cent nose drop solution, is very helpful for either nasal allergies or asthma unless you have heart disease or high blood pressure. Some patients find that ephedrine makes them very restless, especially if they take it in the evening. A quarter of any commonly prescribed sleeping tablet helps to cancel out this action.

These measures frequently will get you through an occasional mild attack. If your allergies cause frequent or severe trouble, your doctor can offer more effective and convenient remedies.

Long-range relief from asthma, hay fever, and allergic sinus or rhinitis. Home measures to remove or trap allergy-causing substances often bring even severe asthma or nasal allergy under control. Dust, pollen, molds and chemicals aggravate every form of breathing passage allergy. These steps often improve or completely relieve allergic distress:

1. Sponge away dust. As a starter, you should get rid of all the accumulated dust (and the pollen which clings to it) from hidden corners of your living quarters. This is one job which you will probably have to get someone to do for you: you can't usually do it yourself without bringing on a disabling allergic attack. A wet sponge or cloth should be the main dirt-removing weapon, since dust cloths only rearrange the dirt without getting rid of it. All drapes, curtains, hangings, and rugs should go into the wash, to the cleaners, or out in the yard for thorough vacuum, home dry cleaning, or soap-and-water cleansing. All pictures, framed mirrors, and the like should be taken down, washed or sponged off, and stored away until Operation Dust-Removal is complete. Go over the furniture—top, bottom, outside, and inside—with an oiled or damp cloth. Vacuum each part of each piece of upholstered furniture, and wipe off each coil of every exposed spring. Remove and sponge or vacuum every item from closets, cupboards, and bookshelves. Get all the dust off of walls and ceilings with thorough sponging. Radiators, hot air registers, and heat ducts are terrific dust-catchers, too.

Once the original job is done, you can probably keep ahead of dust accumulation for yourself for another year. You can use a good vacuum cleaner, although you may have to get someone else to empty the bag. Never sweep or dust dry surfaces: if you want to sweep, soak torn bits of paper in ordinary water and scatter them liberally on the surface to be cleaned. Hit all the dust-catching surfaces in one room or area each week, taking the different parts of the house in rotation. If housecleaning makes you distinctly worse, maybe you can trade chores with someone else in the family.

2. Dispose of dust-catchers and holders. Stuffed toys, big rugs in the bedrooms, and lined drapes which need dry cleaning are dust traps. Washable toys, scatter rugs and light, washable curtains or drapes are usually cheaper than medicines to control your allergies. Or as a last resort, you can simply do without.

3. Settle dust and allergens. You can make most dust and pollen settle out of the air before you breathe it. The less air motion inside your house, the better. That means windows closed tight and doors promptly shut both winter and summer, especially in your own bedroom and living quarters. Oil type furniture polish and oil-containing sweeping compound also help to keep down dust by ensnaring it.

4. Filter out dust and allergens. An air conditioner or electrostatic air cleanser removes many allergens. If you get your doctor to recommend such equipment in writing before you purchase it, cost and maintenance expense usually come off your taxable income, too. Filters for each register are well worthwhile if your heat circulates through ducts.

5. Seal dust-blowing cushions and springs. The biggest single group of dust traps in your home is probably cushions, springs, mattresses and pillows. Every time you sit or lie on such equipment, it acts like a bellows blowing clouds of dust and pollen all around you. The very least you should do is fit all pillows and mattresses in your bedroom with plastic allergy covers. A layer of heavy plastic or oilcloth underneath cotton slipcovers and a sheet of light linoleum tacked to the bottom of each piece of overstuffed furniture may save you a lot of misery, too. You can coat rugs with special dust seal compound. If you have the extra money, foam rubber mattresses and pillows are very comfortable for many allergy sufferers.

6. Seal dust and pollens out of your living quarters. You can't clean all dust and pollen out of attics, cellars, and the great outdoors. But you can often seal these spaces off from your living quarters. A roll of masking tape from any paint or hardware store will seal window cracks, attic doors, and other openings quite thoroughly.

7. Check chemicals. Any chemical substance in your house, from nail polish remover to floor wax to fiberglass insulation (which contains formaldehyde), might be aggravating your allergies. Best first step in finding out which ones you need to replace: take one room each week, and either stay out of it or (in case of your bedroom and such) pack away all the dispensable chemicals in it. If you get better during any one week, try re-introducing one chemical substance every three days until you find all the offenders.

8. No more pets or posies. A cat or canary gives a lot of comfort, but not enough to make it worth the risk for allergy sufferers. Likewise dogs, parakeets, and so on. If you must have something alive around the house, try tropical fish.

Cut flowers and house plants also cause many allergic attacks. Best do without them, at least until your allergies have cleared up. Then you can bring in one plant at a time, so long as new complaints do not appear.

9. Outdoor sports. If you like to swim, three precautions will help: stick to warm water and warm weather, use natural bodies of water instead of chlorinated pools, and avoid calm, unagitated pools. This last precaution is based on the fact that a concentrated layer of pollens and allergens gathers at the surface of a calm pool during the night, and remains until it is dissipated by either wave action or considerable swimming and splashing.

Golf, rides in the country, and other sports involving the great outdoors have considerable risk for allergic people during their seasons. If you must try such sports, take an antihistamine tablet half an hour beforehand.

Cold sores and fever blisters. If you have a tendency toward cold sores, you will get painful blisters which break and leave open sores on your lips with every cold or fever, and sometimes in between. These sometimes will be accompanied by gum sores (see p. 133). You may feel a burning pain and oversensitivity of the spot for a few hours before the blister comes out.

A virus which is present on almost everyone's skin causes these sores. Any time your resistance drops, this virus attacks your tissues. There are two ways to help the situation: by increasing resistance and by soothing the sore when it has already appeared.

Multiple vaccinations. The herpes virus which causes cold sores is apparently a distant cousin of the smallpox virus. If you raise your smallpox immunity to a very high level, some protection against cold sores seems to result. You'll need a doctor's cooperation to try this program, since you can't vaccinate yourself. I usually vaccinate a patient and wait until the vaccination takes, which may take three weeks or so. After the first "take" is well I repeat the vaccination every week for six weeks or so. The repeats never get sore or leave a scar, and the first vaccination only causes a substantial reaction if the person's smallpox immunity has run all the way down (so that vaccination would have been worthwhile even without the cold sores).

It is hard to judge the success of a program which wards off an unpredictable condition like cold sores, but most patients seem to feel that they get help from these vaccinations. If you get cold sores more than two or three times a year, why not give them a try?

Tincture of benzoin. An old Swedish nurse told me about this treatment. She had been using tincture of benzoin as a skin toughener before applying adhesive tape and happened to include a fever blister in the painted area when one of her patients was being bandaged for facial cuts. The victim got so much relief that she has been painting cold sores with benzoin ever since. After trying her discovery, so have I.

Either ordinary or compound tincture of benzoin is available in any drugstore without a prescription. Just paint the cold sore three times a day and let it dry. One caution: blisters which have cloudy fluid in them and burst to form a crusted sore, especially with a thick, crumbly brownish crust, may be impetigo instead of cold sores. Particularly in children (and especially if there are infants in the household, because impetigo is infectious and the very young get terribly sick with it), you should double check apparent cold sores which meet this description.

CHAPTER NINE

Quick Relief for Headache and Tooth, Eye, or Ear Trouble

When a city man with headaches comes to our tranquil lake resorts, he usually leaves his head pain behind. As the last boat pushes off for the bass-haunted lily pads, the happy vacationers seldom see Mr. Resort Owner's careworn face.

"There they go," he's saying to himself. "If the stupid fish don't like the plugs they've brought along, chances are I'll go broke next season!"

So headache remedies don't go begging even in the land of Hiawatha. If anything, the wide open spaces call for more home treatment for headache, toothache, earache, and other miseries. Unless there's a doctor vacationing nearby, North Country people have to depend heavily on their medicine chests. Fortunately, home measures generally give quick and lasting relief.

HEADACHE REMEDIES

Headache often accompanies infection, high blood pressure, kidney trouble, and the like, besides plaguing you independently. You should call your physician promptly whenever headache is accompanied by other signs of disease, such as fever, dizzy spells, nausea, impaired vision, loss of wind on one flight of stairs, swelling of the ankles, or pounding of the heart. Use aspirin, cold cloths, and rest in a darkened room for temporary relief until the doctor comes. For most other headaches you can safely stick with home remedies unless the pain becomes severe or recurs frequently.

Children often complain mainly of headache at the onset of any infection from stomach flu to strep throat. A few specific questions, like "Does it hurt when you swallow?" and "What happens when you take a deep breath?" help you to figure out what the underlying cause might be. Always check for stiff neck, which might point to meningitis or nervous system disease. You might want to hold back on aspirin until you are fairly sure whether you are dealing with a mild virus or a more serious problem. Pain relief might keep any of you from realizing how bad things are. Moreover, making a youngster feel better makes it almost impossible to keep him totally quiet. Since this is often the most important element of cure, your youngster may be better off with enough discomfort to keep him down than with the prolonged and serious consequences of over-activity.

Home remedies for headache. Aspirin is everybody's first thought for headache. Two tablets often do the trick. Another two-tablet dose of aspirin or of aminopyrine (Datril), which works like aspirin without adding to the first dose's side effects, may help if the pain persists after two hours. Buffered aspirin has no real advantage. Excedrin combines aspirin with an ingredient which has both mood-lifting and blood-vessel shrinking effects, and sometimes proves effective.

You can get considerable help from other home measures for several varieties of head pain.

Headaches from fatigue or tension. Most dull, nagging headaches stem from fatigue or tension. Although the pain feels definitely inside, the actual trouble lies in tense scalp muscles and congested veins. In addition to aspirin, these measures often help:

Rest in a darkened room. Rest in a darkened room often helps you to win prompt relief from headache. Patients usually find that they can rest better with no pillow or with a very small pillow or rolled towel placed under the neck. Use your large pillows under your legs, arranged so that the shins are roughly parallel to the floor, and under the lower portion of each arm.

Hot towels. A hot, wet towel relaxes painful scalp muscles and speeds circulation through congested vessels. Fold a towel until it is six to eight layers thick. Dip it in water which is as hot as you can stand without the risk of burning (112° F.). Wring out extra moisture. Cover the wet towel with a dry one to help hold the heat. Dip the towel in hot water every five minutes or so to keep it hot.

Fingertip massage. You can give very effective headache-soothing massage for yourself, although it is still more effective if you can relax completely while someone else strokes your scalp. Start immediately after a hot towel treatment. Use rhythmic strokes with both hands. Sit up with your fingertips pressed gently at the center of your forehead, the fingers limp and the hands parallel to the floor. Brush your fingertips across the forehead, back above the ears to the back of the head. Turn down the neck and follow your jaw line back to the vicinity of the voice box. Repeat rhythmically, with very gentle pressure.

Postural headaches. Although most people picture Minnesotans as rugged outdoorsmen, we have our share of desk workers, too. Secretaries, typists, clerks, and other people whose work involves long periods of sitting erect in almost unchanged posture frequently get dull afternoon headache. These postural headaches stem from the pressure of strained neck muscles on the roots of nerves which lead to the scalp area. Aspirin, heat, and massage give quick relief, but discomfort comes back almost every working day until you take steps to prevent it.

Postural training is the biggest single preventive step. Straighten out the curve of your neck by stretching the back of your head toward the ceiling and simultaneously pushing your chin back and downward as if you were trying to tuck it under your head. Remind yourself continually of this new way of balancing your head for a few days, and soon it will become automatic.

Another helpful measure is to rearrange your desk so that you can do different jobs in slightly different position, at least some of them with your head supported on one hand. If these measures fail, use the neck stretching sling described in Chapter One.

Caffeine withdrawal headaches. Midmorning headaches which plague you on rushed and hectic days may stem partly from missing your usual cup of coffee. Anacin gives quick relief because it contains caffeine, which aspirin does not. Take two tablets at the onset of pain.

Low blood sugar headaches. Steady, dull headaches, which plague you when you wake up in the morning or at the time when your blood sugar sags two or three hours after a sugar-loaded or starchy meal, usually respond quickly to any sugar-containing food. Some patients complain of considerable dizziness with low blood sugar headaches, and others feel weak or sleepy. All these symptoms clear up in five minutes or less if you take a glass of sweetened orange juice or a couple of soft mints. If you are highly subject to such complaints, carry a package of "lifesavers" or some mints at all times. For quick absorption, chew them up instead of sucking them. Try to eat protein food like meat, eggs, or cottage cheese with each meal, don't eat much sweet or starch at one sitting, and make it a point to snack regularly a half hour or so before your usual period of difficulties. With frequent, high protein feedings, your blood sugar probably will never get down to the level that gives you complaints.

Migraine headaches. Although severe migraine certainly calls for a doctor's care, some attacks yield well to home measures. The three main features that help you recognize a migraine attack are preliminary warning sensations, throbbing pain often centered on one side, and frequent nausea or vomiting with attacks. The commonest preliminary warning sensations are shiny spots in front of the eyes, distinctive odors, or crawling skin sensations. The pain may strike quite suddenly or increase gradually over a period of an hour or more. Not quite half of the victims vomit with each attack, but many of the others complain of nausea. Tension kicks off many attacks, so that the soothing tonics you will read about in Chapter Twelve often help.

Strong coffee. Migraines or any other type of throbbing headaches usually stem from engorged blood vessels. Strong coffee helps to shrink those vessels. One or two cups of strong coffee usually do enough good through this effect to make up for their jitters-spurring action. In severe attacks with nausea and vomiting, you sometimes can get relief by cooling a cup of strong coffee and taking it very slowly as an enema, retaining it as long as possible.

Ice bags. Ice also helps to shrink engorged blood vessels. Ice bags should be padded with a dry towel or a knitted or flannel bag to prevent ice burns. If you do not have a rubber ice bag, a plastic refrigerator bag works fairly well. Apply the ice for 20 minutes at a time, allowing the skin to rest for at least 10 minutes between applications.

Aspirin. Use aspirin, not A.P.C. or other compounds in conjunction with the coffee cure. Three tablets help dull caffeine jitters and fight pain. If you weigh 150 pounds or more, take four tablets for an initial dose.

Rest. Rest in a darkened room helps migraine and other throbbing headaches considerably. Some of my patients have even found eye shades worthwhile.

Diet. During a migraine headache, most patients do not want any food. Warm broth, moderately chilled (not ice cold) ginger ale, or juice may sit fairly well. Avoid very hot and very cold foods for 24 hours.

Prescription medicines. Besides remedies for migraine itself, you might ask your doctor about anti-nauseants and nerve settlers which make fine supplements to other migraine control measures.

Eyestrain headaches. Eyestrain can cause either throbbing or steady headaches, as well as nausea, dulled concentration, and dizziness. Aspirin and rest usually give quick relief. You can usually avoid further trouble through these measures:

Light your work well, at least one-fifth with indirect or bounced light to avoid harsh shadows.

Turn your workbench or chair away from patches of gloom or glare. Excessive contrast greatly increases eye fatigue. This same principle demands some soft light in the room while you watch TV.

Sit up with your work or reading matter held straight in front of you.

If eyestrain headaches continue, have your eyes examined to see if new glasses would help.

HOME MEASURES FOR TOOTH TROUBLES

You can usually relieve a toothache with home measures, at least until you can get further dental care. You can cut down the number of cavities requiring expensive and uncomfortable care. You can slow or curb the tooth socket and gum disorders which cause more lost teeth than all other dental diseases put together.

How to relieve a toothache. Aspirin and well-padded ice bags give some relief from cavity-caused toothache, which you can spot by recalling recent twinges of pain when eating sweets and by finding a brownish or dead-white crater in the shiny enamel of the painful tooth. These further measures are worthwhile:

Oil of cloves. Mild toothache often responds to warm oil of cloves. Pour a little oil into a teaspoon. Warm it with a match. Dab it onto the cavity area with a toothpick or wooden matchstick.

Zinc oxide-oil poultice. Oil alone will not seal larger cavities. Mix up a thick paste of zinc oxide powder and oil of cloves for these. Press a glob of this mixture into the cavity area with your fingertip, then clean off the excess from the surrounding area with the blunt end of a toothpick.

Abscessed teeth. Probably the main thing to do about abscessed teeth is to recognize them so that you don't suffer along for several extra days. A swollen jaw, throbbing pain and some fever usually mean abscess. You can usually spot abscess without swelling or fever by tapping on each tooth in turn with some small metal object when you get pain. An abscess hurts when you tap on the tooth from which it took its start. You can usually get relief for a few hours until you see your dentist by taking two teaspoonfuls of paregoric and full doses of aspirin. A well-padded ice bag also helps.

Soft teeth. If you have a tendency to form cavities very easily, you can probably save yourself considerable misery and expense with these three measures:

Flouride coating. Although fluoridated water does little or nothing for adults, you can harden your tooth enamel at any age by painting it with fluoride. Your dentist can apply strong solutions to your teeth. A safe home corrective for soft teeth is toothpaste which contains stannous fluoride. Brush thoroughly enough to work the lather across every surface of every tooth daily for about a one-third reduction in cavities.

Diet. A low sugar diet for six to eight weeks can cut your rate of cavity formation for about two years. You can use sucaryl or other calorie-free sugar substitutes to make this program easier. Avoid between-meals eating, sugar-sweetened beverages and desserts for eight weeks, then count the savings in your dental bills.

After-meal mouth rinse. You can cut the number of acid-forming germs in your mouth very substantially by rinsing out your mouth. Take a mouthful of water at the end of each meal and after each between-meals snack or sweetened beverage. Swish the water around your mouth and between your teeth several times, then swallow it or spit it out. This simple technique removes as much as ninety per cent of the germ-breeding food residues from your mouth, and substantially reduces cavity formation. It is especially worthwhile if you cannot brush your teeth after each meal.

Home measures against periodontitis. You can substantially reduce infection of the gums and tooth sockets, which causes a tremendous number of teeth to be lost, with simple home measures. Periodontitis shows up as soreness or tenderness of the gums, sometimes with bleeding. In some cases, loosening of the teeth and tenderness on chewing are the first warning signs. Even if the disease has reached the stage where teeth are quite loose, however, you can often get them to tighten up again with proper care.

Fingertip massage. You usually have to start fingertip massage gradually, since periodontitis makes your gums tender. Begin with one minute of massage twice a day. Moisten the tip of your index finger and reach back inside your cheek but outside of your teeth. Press your fingertip firmly against the upper gum as high up and as far back as possible. Slide the fingertip down toward the teeth. Relax the pressure and return your finger to a spot above the next tooth or space. Press and slide the fingertip downward again. Continue in this manner all the way around the outside of the upper gum. Follow a similar procedure with the lower gum, massaging firmly with strokes beginning far down on the gum and sliding toward the tooth crests. Open the mouth wide. Use small circular motions to massage the inside surface of the gums. If you have a tendency to gag, pant in and out while working far back in the mouth. After finishing fingertip massage chew on a moderately heavy rubber band for two minutes or so as you go about your business, being especially careful to chew with all available grinders. Don't spare slightly loose or tender teeth.

Toothbrush massage. After two or three weeks of fingertip massage, you may want to start using toothbrush massage, too. Toothbrush strokes should always start well up on the gum and sweep downward toward the tooth points. Ten strokes in each area with a firm brush stimulates circulation considerably.

Gum sores. If you are subject to gum and mouth sores when you are tired or have an upset stomach, you know just how painful they can be. Ordinary sores with a whitish coating and rim of reddish tissue respond well to home measures. If the whitish portion looks leathery, the edges seem heaped-up, or the sores do not heal inside two weeks, see your doctor.

Silver nitrate. If you treat mouth sores right away, you can often shorten their course considerably with silver nitrate. I usually moisten the tip of a cotton-tipped applicator with 10% silver nitrate solution, which you can get at any drugstore without a prescription, and hold it in gentle contact with the ulcer for 5 or 10 seconds, then get the patient to rinse out his mouth with a little water. If you try this technique, use sparing amounts of the solution and keep it right in the sore, since it may otherwise harm the normal surrounding tissue slightly. Keep the silver nitrate separate from other medicines and in a place that is safe from children, since it is quite poisonous.

Gly-Oxide(R). This patent medicine remedy is available in any drugstore without a prescription and works rather well for canker sores, gum sores, irritation. from denture rub and so forth. It is packaged in an applicator-top bottle, which makes it easy to apply directly to the sore. Put it on four times a day, following the package directions.

Salt water mouthwash. Whether you apply silver nitrate or not, you can keep down soreness and secondary infection by washing your mouth out thoroughly with mild salt solution three or four times a day. Half a teaspoonful of table salt to a glass of warm water is very soothing.

Gum boils. A sore spot or area on the gums which is red and swollen may be a gum boil. Sometimes a tooth abscess will also drain this way. Aspirin and an ice bag may give temporary relief, but you almost always need some help from a dentist to clear up these conditions.

WATCH FOR DANGER SIGNALS

You can care for many eye troubles for yourself with well-chosen home measures, but you should first check for evidence of possibly serious conditions before you try any treatment on inflamed or painful eyes. See your doctor promptly if any of these signs show up:

Pain in the eyes, over the eyes, or in the back of the head. Abrupt increase in pressure within the eye may cause intense pain. Smoldering cases of glaucoma cause less violent discomfort, which may come and go. Pain starts or becomes worse when the pupils grow larger: in darkness or during an emotional upheaval.

Halos around lights. A rainbow band around street lamps on a clear night may be due to early glaucoma. If you see your doctor promptly, you'll probably be cured without operation and with no loss of vision.

Abrupt worsening of vision. After age 40, your eyes should not change size and shape enough to make you need new glasses more than every two to five years. If either your distant or your close vision becomes notably more blurred within a six-month period, check with your eye doctor to see whether glaucoma or eye changes due to diabetes, high blood pressure, or hardening of the arteries might be responsible. Your doctor can give you help with all of these problems.

Eyes that thrive in gloom. If you see much better in a dimly lit room or with dark glasses, the reason may be a cataract. Cataracts are cloudy spots in one of your eye's light-gathering parts. They often start in the center of the pupil. When you are in a brightly lit room, your pupil becomes smaller so that the still-clear parts of your eye's light-gathering apparatus are blanked out. Result: dim vision in well-lit rooms, better vision in gloom.

A magenta band. If infection or injury involves the clear window into the eye or the deeper tissues, a dusky magenta band about a quarter of an inch wide shows up on the white of the eye around the iris. Sometimes you have to look very closely to distinguish this from the overlay of pinkish inflammation involving the whole white of the eye, which comes with any condition involving rubbing or congestion. If you can't be sure, let your doctor put in some drops which blank out this confusing overlay.

HOME CARE FOR EYE TROUBLES

How to remove a cinder from your eye. When something gets into your eye, tears form immediately to help wash it out. You can aid this normal body mechanism, use other washing techniques, or get someone to remove the cinder for you by flipping the lid. Here are detailed directions:

Aiding your tears. As soon as something flies into your eye, you should close the lid gently and place your fingertip on the lashes. Press straight down along the front of your cheek bone, so that the upper and lower lids both pull slightly away from the eyeball and make a pocket in front of the eye. Let this reservoir fill with tears. Without moving your finger, snap the upper lid open. Then move your finger and allow the lower lid to recoil. Usually the cinder will float out with the accumulated tears.

Eyewashes. Stir one teaspoonful of boric acid powder into a glass of warm water. If any powder is left, let it settle to the bottom and be careful not to get it into your eye. Fill an eyedropper with the overlying clear fluid. Lean your head back and hold both lids of the affected eye as far open as possible with your thumb and forefinger. Squirt the solution into the eye. Repeat three or four times if necessary

Lid flipping. If milder measures fail, you need to get help from a friend or member of your family. Have your helper carefully search for the cinder on your eyeball by pulling the lower lid down. If he is unable to locate it, the cinder is probably inside your upper lid. Look down without closing your eye. Have your helper grasp your upper eyelashes between his thumb and forefinger. He can then press the side of a pencil point or a small key straight into the lid about an eighth of an inch above the lid margin. The cartilage pad inside the lid, which is perhaps a half inch wide, will flip down over the pupil. By stretching the skin of the lid slightly from the sides, your helper can keep the lid cartilage from flipping back into place while he dabs at the cinder with the corner of a clean handkerchief. If the lid fails to flip back as soon as he lets go, you can replace it easily by opening the eye extra wide with your thumb and forefinger.

Tired eyes, TV eyes. If you are subject to eye fatigue, rest breaks may help. At the end of the first paragraph of every fourth page while you are reading, stop for a moment, let your head nod, and close your eyes. You will feel the tiredness flow out of them over a period of a few seconds, after which you can start reading again. Use commercials for eye rest instead of household chores or conversation when you are watching TV. You will find that a few seconds' break gives your eyes a fresh start.

Salt water rinsing. If you suffer from eye fatigue in spite of brief rest breaks, try salt water rinsing. Let some water stand overnight in an open basin so that all the chlorine escapes. Add a level teaspoonful of table salt to a pint of water. Be sure all the crystals are thoroughly dissolved, and that there is no dirt in the solution. Keep it in a stoppered bottle in a fairly cool place. When your eyes become very fatigued, put some of the moderately cool solution in an eye cup and wash your eyes with it, each for a few moments.

Bloodshot or burning eyes, including pink-eye. Burning, irritated, bloodshot eyes call for mildly astringent drops or ointment. The form of mild eye inflammation which spreads from person to person also yields to these medications. Here is the formula I usually recommend, which druggists in some states can supply without a prescription:

> Zinc sulfate ¼ per cent.
> Saturated solution of boric acid 1 oz.

Put two drops in each eye three or four times a day. Like many potent eye drops, this burns when you first put it in. Don't be alarmed: the burning will quickly subside.

Some patients prefer to use an eye ointment instead of drops. Zinc sulfate ½ per cent works quite well. If you try to put in an eye ointment for yourself, lie down and hold the lids apart. Brace the tube-squeezing thumb against the bridge of your nose. Squirt an amount of ointment equivalent to a small green pea in the inner corner of your eye. In a few seconds, it will melt and spread across the eye. Then you can release the lids and wipe off the surplus ointment with a clean handkerchief.

Sties. Hot cloths help to bring sties to a head. Mild antiseptic ointment helps to keep the germs from one sty from ultimately causing another.

Hot cloths. Fold an ordinary washcloth to four layers' thickness. Dip in water which is as hot as is comfortable (112 degrees) and wring partially dry. Apply to eye, and cover with a dry towel to help hold the heat. Change as often as necessary to keep the cloth hot for twenty minutes.

Antiseptic ointment. If you can get an antiseptic eye ointment like Bacitracin or Furacin without a prescription in your state, it usually helps. Otherwise, old-fashioned yellow oxide of mercury does fairly well. Apply in the inner corner of the eye three times a day. Let it melt and spread across before releasing the lids. If sties occur frequently or fail to yield to these measures, best check with your eye doctor.

HOW TO MANAGE COMMON EAR PROBLEMS FOR YOURSELF

You can probably control some forms of earache and infection, most accumulation of wax, and the commonest varieties of itching, irritated ear canals without a doctor's help. You should suspect disease for which a doctor's prompt care is probably worthwhile when these signs are present:

1. Running ears.
2. Persistent ringing in the ears.
3. Earache accompanied by fever or hearing loss.

Otherwise, home measures are usually worth a try.

The chewing gum cure. An earache often comes from stopped-up air passages. The tube through which air moves into the middle ear space starts near your adenoids. A cold can puff up these tissues until they block off this air tube. Some of the air inside the ear cavity then soaks into your system, leaving a vacuum which sucks back on the drum, stretching it painfully.

Some of your muscles attach to your ear's inner air tube, and certain chewing motions tend to pull the tube open or milk air bubbles through it. That is the basis for the chewing gum cure's effectiveness. An ordinary stick of gum won't do the trick because the movements required have to be quite wide An adult should chew three pieces of bubble gum (a child should chew two) for an hour or so at a time two or three times a day. If a stopped air tube is causing the trouble, the ear will usually either "pop" or "crackle" as air comes into it.

This cure is also very effective for the feeling of fullness and discomfort after an airplane ride or a trip over the mountains. Even when you don't have a cold, rapid changes in altitude can create a pressure problem which collapses the ear's pressure equalization tube. Chewing a big wad of gum often opens things up.

Even without fever or throbbing, earache can be due to infection, especially if nose-blowing and sneezing have driven germs up into the ear cavity. Don't stick with the chewing gum cure too long under these circumstances, and check frequently for fever or hearing loss which point toward conditions for which a physician's care should give prompt help.

Home remedies for simple earache. For earaches which come on after wind exposure or other irritation, try these measures:

Ear drops. Olive oil, sweet oil, or dehydrated glycerin gives considerable relief when used as ear drops. Warm a dropperful in a dry spoon, using a match or candle. Test on the back of your hand. Lie on your side with the bad ear up and flood the ear canal with the warm drops. Apply a well padded hot water bottle over the ear to help hold the warmth.

Pain-easing medicines. You probably should stick to aspirin alone instead of using the paregoric-aspirin mixture if you do not plan to see a doctor right away, so that if the pain persists or grows worse you will be aware that all is not going well.

How to keep ear wax from piling up. You can keep ear wax from accumulating in your ear canal by applying home measures. You can put wax-softening solutions into the ear canal with perfect safety (unless your doctor has told you to keep all fluid out of your ears because of a perforated eardrum). Once the wax is soft, the slight back and forth motion of the ear canal that occurs with chewing will usually milk it out of your ears.

Homemade wax-softening solution. You can make and use your own wax-softening solution. Mix three drops of any modern liquid dishwashing detergent with one teaspoonful of warm water. Lie on your left side. Put about half of the solution into your right ear. Let it soak in for about one minute. Turn on your right side, holding a handkerchief over the ear opening to soak up excess solution as it runs out. Put the rest of the solution into the left ear, and let it soak in for one minute. Repeat the whole procedure three times a day for three successive days whenever wax begins to accumulate. If the wax has not worked out after three days, a gentle stream of warm water from an all-rubber ear syringe will often wash it free.

Boils in the ear canals. If you get severe throbbing or steady pain in the ears without hearing loss or fever, your problem is sometimes a boil in the ear canal. The skin is tied to the underlying cartilage so tightly that very little swelling can occur, yet the pressure of infection causes considerable pain. Main tip-off: ear canal infections hurt when you move the outer ear up and down, while inner ear infections do not.

Ichthyol wick. Old fashioned ichthyol ointment helps considerably for ear boils. The easiest way to keep it in contact with the sore is with a thin gauze wick. Cut an 8'' length of one-inch roller gauze bandage lengthwise in half and work it around in a bit of ichthyol ointment until it is thoroughly impregnated. Double one end of it over a cotton tipped applicator and insert half an inch into the ear canal. Hold the wick in place with the blunt end of a toothpick while you withdraw the applicator. Double another fold of wick in front of the ear opening and push it back into the ear with the applicator. Continue until the ear canal is snugly packed with wick.

A new product called Cresatin is probably better than ichthyol, but at the moment most druggists can only sell it on prescription.

Itching or discomfort in the ear canals. Smoldering fungus or bacterial infection of the ear canals commonly causes considerable itching and discomfort. If this condition is severe, you should probably get medical help with it. For mild cases, try this technique:

Burow's wick. Gently work a piece of absorbent cotton back into the ear canal. Get an ounce or more of Burow's solution 1:1000 from your druggist. Keep the wick wet with the solution all through the day and night. Change wicks daily, allowing the ear canal to dry out for an hour or so.

Castellani's paint. If Burow's solution fails, you might try Castellani's paint in exactly the same way. This material stains clothing, linens and everything in sight. Best keep a puff of clean dry cotton tucked in the ear on top of the saturated wick to keep down the mess.

CHAPTER TEN

How to Control Skin Allergies, Rashes, and Infections

Skin trouble is an assault by four horsemen: itching, soreness, aggravation, and pain. Yet I have seen patients who endured this misery for years without even seeking relief. Such futile suffering! Most of these victims could cure themselves in their own homes, with almost no expense, if they only knew what measures to take. The rest could almost always get at least temporary relief from home measures. Yet I have seen my good Minnesota patients itching and squirming without attempting to take these easy steps toward relief.

HOW TO FIGHT SKIN IRRITATIONS AND ALLERGIES

Chemical irritation causes many more visits to a skin specialist's office than any one skin disease. You can very frequently soothe those irritations right in your own home, with little or no expense. Furthermore, you can often discover what substances cause your trouble and eliminate them for permanent cure.

Sensitive skin. No matter what harsh chemical irritates your skin, you get the same complaints and changes, and need the same home remedies. Even if you mistake some other skin disease for skin sensitivity, properly chosen measures will usually prove highly effective, or at least harmless. Whenever you have skin irritation which is not so severe as to drive you to a doctor for powerful prescription aid, try these soothing remedies:

Weeping or blistered skin. Home remedies for blistered or weeping sores usually prove worthwhile unless pussy matter or thick, crumbling crusts point toward impetigo or similar infection. Wet applications rather than lotions or ointments are the safest home treatment for irritation-caused weeping, blisters, or cracks.

Soothing soaks. Two tablespoonfuls of Burow's solution to one pint of water at room temperature is the best remedy. Boric acid solution, one tablespoonful of powder to the pint, is second best for adults (but is not safe for children). A level teaspoonful of table salt to one pint of water or full strength cow's milk makes satisfactory soaks if you have nothing else on hand. If the dermatitis involves parts easily immersed such as hands, feet, or elbows, soak for 10 to 15 minutes at least four times daily. For other body parts, apply cloths wet with soothing solution for twenty minutes at least four times a day. With very severe rashes, you may want to use these measures still more frequently.

Skin healing baths. Severe itching of widespread body parts calls for oatmeal baths. These usually give relief for eight hours or so, and speed healing of almost any type of dermatitis. Follow these directions:

> Boil two cups of slow-cooking oatmeal in two quarts of water for fifteen minutes. Fill your bathtub halfway with moderately warm water. Hold a piece of light cotton or fairly fine cheesecloth over the bathtub and pour the oatmeal into it. A light cotton sack or bag works very well. The cloth should strain the oatmeal out and allow the fluid to drain through into the tub. Gather the edges of the cloth and tie above the oatmeal with string. Now get into the tub. Use the oatmeal bag as a washcloth to pat the worst itching areas, and slosh it around in the bath water at intervals. Soak in the soothing solution for about 20 minutes.

Colloid baths. If your skin eruption seems likely to last more than a few days, you can get the benefit of oatmeal baths without the bother by using the purified oatmeal colloid, sold in your drugstore under the trade name "Aveeno." Use two cupfuls to a tub of water, and soak yourself for 20 minutes as often as your complaints require.

Soothing measures for red or raw skin eruptions. Skin irritations which are too mild to blister or crack usually yield to lotions or pastes. Most patchy, itching eruptions fall in this group.

Lotion. You can get zinc oxide lotion, which is very soothing for most skin lesions, without a prescription. Buy a small bottle of glycerin at the same time for use in removing cakes or crusts left by the lotion at the end of the day.

Pastes and ointments. If the irritated area is dry, scaly, or harsh-feeling, pastes and ointments work better than lotion. Lassar's paste requires no prescription, and is very soothing. Boric acid or zinc oxide ointments also help mildly irritated skin.

Home correctives for common skin sensitivities. You can usually cure skin irritation for good by using suitable substitutes for the substances that have been causing your trouble. The big trick is to identify the troublemakers. Keep track of when the rash flares and fades and watch what objects come in contact with the affected area. Then decide which might be offenders by keeping these points in mind:

1. Dermatitis usually flares inside 24 hours of contact with the offending irritant. However, the abruptness of the flare does not mean that it occurs immediately after contact. One of my good farm women, for instance, developed a rash that itched and burned abruptly almost every evening after supper. When we finally discovered the source of her difficulty, it proved to be allergy to the chicken mash she spread by hand every morning, twelve to eighteen hours before the rash flared.

2. Dermatitis often develops suddenly from exposure to a substance that you have used previously without harmful effects. One of my patients had been in the baking trade for 24 years before he developed a rash, which we nevertheless proved was due to flour. A great many patients who learn the cause of their trouble only after several visits to a doctor say: "Well, I would have figured that out for myself, only I've used the same stuff for years without trouble."

3. Dermatitis usually starts in the general vicinity of the spot touched by the offending substances, but there are several notable exceptions. The thick skin of the palm of the hand seldom becomes inflamed, so that inflammation of the back of the hand, wrist and lower arms often occurs from substances most of whose contact is with the palm. Fingernail polish frequently causes inflammation of the eyelids. Any dermatitis which becomes severe can spread far beyond the area of actual chemical irritation.

Let's see how these principles have helped several skin sufferers:

1. A housewife found that her blistered hands got worse every Friday. Since she cleaned house on Thursday, she soon traced her trouble to furniture polish.

2. A printer's face bumps got almost well by Monday morning, became troublesome again during the week. He ultimately found that he was sensitive to the brand of soap his boss provided.

3. A bank clerk whose hobby was photography came to work every Monday morning with red, raw hands until he learned that his skin reacted to one of the chemicals he used in his weekend darkroom work.

All of these victims cured themselves by applying the simple facts about skin sensitivity. Couldn't you do the same?

Specific skin irritations. Some eruptions due to sensitive skin are so common that you can take a short cut to quick cure if you know about them. Here are specific directions for spotting and curing these common skin sensitivities:

Soap-burnt hands. Dry, rough, cracking skin on the hands usually comes from soap or detergents. More severe, weeping, or blistering eruption of the backs or sides of the fingers and hands may also be due to soap. Ideal solution: avoid doing dishes, laundry, or floor-scrubbing, at least until the rash is clear. Second best: wear lined rubber gloves or a pair of white cotton gloves with rubber gloves over them until your skin is clear. For continued protection, try a silicone protective lotion or cream such as Covicone, which you can get at any drugstore without a prescription. Apply three times a day for one week, twice a day for one week, and daily thereafter. Most patients find this as effective as rubber gloves and much less clumsy. For handwashing, super-bland detergents like pHisoderm work well. Nonperfumed bland soap like Ivory or Swan may prove safe after your hands have thoroughly healed.

Itching scalp If itching scalp plagues you, or if you have a rash along the tops or backs of the ears and on your neck, shampoo chemicals may be at fault. One way to find out: clean your hair with the raw egg method for one month.

Egg shampoo. Beat two or three raw eggs, wet the hair with warm water, and rub in the beaten eggs thoroughly with the tips of your fingers. Rinse thoroughly with lukewarm water. Follow with a vinegar rinse, made from one teaspoonful of white vinegar in one quart of lukewarm water. Brush thoroughly while the hair is drying.

Saponified coconut oil. If you have only a normal degree of itching, you might want to try a special form of liquid soap as a shampoo. Saponified coconut oil, obtained from any pharmacy, is much gentler, more effective, and cheaper than most commercial shampoos. Many of my patients find it highly satisfactory for regular scalp cleansing.

Laundry detergent rash. Dry, red-pepper-granule dermatitis of the back and upper arms is often due to laundry detergent. The clothing clings in these areas. Perspiration provides a perfect bridge for chemicals to cross in reaching the skin. You can cure this condition quickly by washing clothes in bland soap powder such as Ivory Snow and rinsing them three times in soft water.

Cosmetic rash. When I ask a lady with a skin rash about cosmetics, she usually says: "But I don't use any." Most people take simple beauty aids like lipstick, cleansing cream, toilet water and nail polish for granted. Yet these quite commonly cause skin trouble. Most women with blemishes or rash should eliminate all beauty aids, perfumed soaps and shampoos, nail polish and deodorants for a two week period. If the rash clears, they should resume beauty aids one at a time with a week or more lag between new agents until they find the offenders. Usually, different brands or specially compounded cosmetics will fill the beauty bill without causing further trouble.

Workman's eruption. Most people encounter harsh chemicals of some sort in the course of their work. Cutting oils, cement dust, harsh solvents, and cleaning agents are the commonest offenders on a mile-long list. If you have skin trouble which improves during vacations, your work is probably responsible. Under workmen's compensation laws, your employer usually has to pay for any care you need, so you might as well see a doctor. Moreover, you need the doctor's certificate that work caused your trouble before you can settle your claim.

Rash from medicines. Probably the commonest form of sensitive-skin rash which you can control with home measures stems from your attempts to get and keep well. Every kind of medicine from aspirin tablets and vitamin capsules to skin lotions and ointments can sometimes cause skin rash. You can control or avoid this difficulty by following these rules:

1. Whenever you get a rash, eliminate all self-prescribed or non-essential medicines, including vitamin pills, laxatives, sleeping pills, and aspirin. If your doctor has prescribed medicines which you should continue because of some serious condition, call him up and ask him whether there is any chance that the medicine could be causing your rash.

2. If an abruptly appearing rash persists for more than two weeks or gets worse in spite of treatment, eliminate all ointments and applications (including any your doctor has prescribed). Use Burow's solution soaks or cloths, which are always safe, to keep your disorder under control. If medications have been prolonging or aggravating your condition, you should note an improvement inside two days.

3. Treat skin ailments more gently the worse they seem to be. Use milder soaks instead of stronger ointments for persistent or highly troublesome skin ailments. Over-strong medicines drive more patients to skin specialists than any single disease. You can frequently keep yourself from requiring expensive specialized services for this reason.

Here are two instructive examples:

H. G. developed an itchy, reddish blotch on the back of his left hand. His druggist suggested 5% ammoniated mercury ointment. After a week the rash seemed somewhat worse, so H. G. bought some stronger ointment—10% ammoniated mercury. Two weeks later, H. G. went to his doctor with blistering and redness extending almost up to his left elbow, and some rash of the back of the right hand. Key step to quick cure: omitting any further ammoniated mercury ointment.

M. T. had always used Whitfield's ointment for his athlete's foot, with excellent results. When he developed an unusually severe case with open cracks between his toes and burning blisters, he figured Whitfield's would do the trick. It burned like fire in the open cracks, but M. T. used it anyway. After ten days, his feet were so bad that he couldn't get to work any longer. On his wife's advice he switched to Burow's solution soaks. In two days, he was virtually well.

HOW TO CONTROL SKIN INFECTIONS WITH SIMPLE HOME CARE

You can control many small skin infections with simple home remedies and care. Ingrown hairs, boils, beginning infection beside the fingernail, mild festering, athlete's foot, and scabies frequently yield to proper home treatment. Here are several pointers for recognizing and dealing with these common problems:

Boils, ingrown hair, and infected sores. With a little help, your body can almost always fight off the germs that cause boils and minor skin infections. It does this by pouring germ-devouring white blood cells into the area. These white blood cells soon pile up in the form of pus and matter, which works to the skin surface. You can aid this natural method of body defense in several important ways:

1. Hot soaks or wet cloths. Heat helps to open up blood vessels in the infected area, lets more germ-devouring white blood cells get to the scene, and makes infections come to a head much more quickly. If the sore is on a hand or foot where you can soak it, put the whole part down in water as hot as is completely comfortable (about 112 degrees, measured with a candy thermometer). Otherwise use a towel that's folded to six or eight thicknesses and dipped in hot water. Wring out the excess water and cover with a dry towel or piece of plastic. Switch to a freshly-dipped towel as often as necessary. Whether you soak or use cloths, continue the heat for 20 minutes at least four times a day.

2. How to open a pointed up sore. Pus or matter works its way toward the surface of your skin. It usually takes a day or two to stretch the skin and burst through. Once you can see yellow or white pus welling up in an infected sore, you can speed healing by opening it. The transparent skin at the point of a sore is dead tissue anyway, and ultimately will give away.

The best home method for opening a sore is with a flamed needle. First, clean the sore and the nearby skin with rubbing alcohol. Then pass the needle through a flame several times. Let the needle cool without touching anything. Hold the needle almost level with the skin. Push the tip along just under the point of the sore, but always within the transparent area. Lift up to break through the skin. Let the pus well up, perhaps pressing *very gently* on the area. Do not try to squeeze the pus out—more hot soaks will draw it out more safely and comfortably. Clean the surrounding skin again with alcohol. Put on a bandage. Use further hot soaks, right through the bandage.

3. Favor the infected part. You can help to heal an infection and limit its spread simply by resting the part. If you have any festering sore, every muscle you move in the vicinity milks some germs into the surrounding area. A big bandage that holds the part still and reminds you not to use it will speed your recovery a great deal. If bandaging isn't practical, favor the infected part as much as you can.

4. Germicidal cleansing. After each soak or at least four times a day, you should wipe off the whole area surrounding any infected sore with rubbing alcohol. At least once a day, you should definitely take a thorough shower with antiseptic-containing surgical soap such as Gamophene, obtainable at any drugstore without prescription. If the sore is located in your armpit or in another area where skin surfaces rub together, apply 5% ammoniated mercury ointment, which also requires no prescription, to the surrounding area twice a day. These precautions will help to keep the hordes of still-potent germs which stream out with the pus from infecting other nearby skin glands and perpetuating your problem. To cite a case:

"I've had so many boils in my armpits," Mrs. Simpson complained. "Eight or ten every year now, for the past twelve years."

Mrs. Simpson had tried countless kinds of medicine. She had given up deodorants and stopped shaving her armpits. Still she suffered misery from her boils. A program based on germicidal cleansing stopped all that. Mrs. Simpson washed her armpits thoroughly with surgical soap and wiped them with rubbing alcohol three times a day. Only one more boil appeared. While it was draining, she smeared 5 per cent ammoniated mercury ointment on all of the skin in the area to keep germs from getting into nearby glands. She washed her armpits with alcohol six times a day. From that time forth, she never had another boil.

Infection around a fingernail. Infections at the margin of the fingernails cause a great deal of pain. You can often stop such an infection for yourself without a doctor's help by prompt action.

Hot soaks. As soon as infection causes redness, throbbing pain, and slight swelling at the base or side of the nail, you should start using hot soaks. Soak the whole finger for twenty minutes at least four times a day in water which is as hot as you can stand without burning (112 degrees). This helps to draw the infection and get it ready to drain

Drainage. You can often drain an infection around the fingernail before it starts to point up. Immediately after a hot soak, work the tip of a small scissors blade gently under the cuticle beside your infection. Gently lift the tip straight up to pull the cuticle away from the underlying nail. Work it in a little farther, and lift again. Repeat until matter wells up, or until further manipulation becomes painful. Do this every time you soak the finger for a day or so. If a drop or two of pus or matter does not drain out before two days have passed, best see a doctor.

Prevention. Housewives get eight times as many infections around the fingernails as office workers. The whole family's mouth germs wind up in the dishwater where they get a perfect whack at mother's fingers. This is one risk any woman can easily avoid. Just rinse your hands in a fresh stream of water for a few seconds after you dump the dishpan.

How to cure athlete's foot with home measures. You can usually control athlete's foot for yourself, without a doctor's aid. Itching, cracking, and peeling between the toes usually come from simple athlete's foot. Small blisters filled with cloudy fluid may spread to the base of the toes and the instep. Here's how to rid yourself of this disease:

Soaks. Heal open blisters or cracks with soaks before you use ointment on your athlete's foot. Potassium permanganate works well. It stains, so use an old basin or pot for soaking. Crush a five grain tablet thoroughly and dissolve it in one quart of water. Be sure the tablet is completely dissolved, because undissolved fragments will burn your skin. Soak your feet ten minutes every two hours. The soaks will turn your toenails brown, but this is a harmless color change. Permanganate tablets are very poisonous, so keep them in a safe place and flush leftover supplies down the toilet when you are well. Two to four days of soaking usually does the trick.

Ointments. If you have no open blisters or cracks, or if you have healed them with soaks, undecenylic acid ointment is your best bet. Apply it twice daily for at least one week after signs of athlete's foot have disappeared. In a few cases, undecenylic acid fails. Then you can use half strength Whitfield's ointment. Do not use full strength Whitfield's, which is too strong for many people's skin.

If ointments cause irritation, or if your condition fails to improve, see your doctor.

Sock sterilization. Athlete's foot germs can live for several months nestled in shoe leather or between the threads of your socks. By sterilizing your socks after each wearing and changing them every day, you can usually keep athlete's foot from coming back. The water you use in your own washing machine or in a self-help laundry is not hot enough to kill these germs. Either brief boiling or a trip to a commercial laundry (which uses water at 180 degrees) makes socks safe.

Measures to avoid reinfection. Once you know that you are susceptible to athlete's foot, you can save yourself a lot of misery by taking steps to avoid reinfection. Be sure that everyone in your household with even a trace of athlete's foot takes treatment at once. Take special precautions when you use a public shower or bath. Dry well between your toes: that prevents nine cases out of ten. If hazard is very high, as in the men's shower at work, use foot clogs and rub your feet with alcohol just before drying.

Psoriasis. The scaly, dry patches of psoriasis show up most frequently on the elbows, knees, and at the hairline. Fortunately, this unsightly state does not disfigure the face or cause unbearable itching and discomfort. Most victims have had trouble since their teens, and have asked doctors about the condition often enough to know exactly what is wrong with them and that no lasting cure is presently available. However, these simple home techniques usually give considerable improvement:

Ultraviolet ray. If your psoriasis tends to get better in the summertime, you will probably improve with ultraviolet ray baths. You will get the best results with an ultraviolet lamp which has a quartz tube rather than a glass one, since the most beneficial rays cannot pass through glass. A glass sunlight bulb is better than nothing, though. Several of my patients are in the habit of taking a sunbath while shaving and performing their morning toilet, which helps to make the treatments regular and still saves considerable time. During the summer, you can replace lamp treatments with natural sun baths.

Ultraviolet through tar ointment. One of the most effective measures for most psoriasis victims is the combination ointment-ultraviolet treatment. For this treatment, spread a thin coat of

Taralba ointment over the scaly patches of psoriasis, then take a sunbath treatment right through the ointment. Either natural sunlight or ultraviolet light does well.

Ointment alone. A few psoriasis victims find that they get worse in the summertime or after sunbathing. These people should carefully protect themselves from sun, coating their psoriasis sores with a little petroleum jelly when protection with clothing is not practical. An ordinary tar ointment helps most smoldering lesions. Very thick, heaped up plaques sometimes respond to a thorough mixture of three parts Taralba with one part Whitfield's ointment. Tegrin and Mazon ointments are good trade preparations.

Bland measures. When psoriasis shows signs of becoming rapidly worse, with new spots appearing, old spots spreading, or considerable itching and discomfort, you should usually omit any tar or ultraviolet treatment. At this stage, zinc oxide ointment and soothing oatmeal baths often help. Your doctor's advice will prove worthwhile, too.

The itch. You would think a disorder linked with crowding and body contact would be rare in Minnesota. But North Country folks huddle together for warmth and rub elbows in congeniality. North Country children grapple on the beaches in the summer and on the hockey rink most of the year. North Country homes and schools always have a crowded coatrack or mud room filled with a jumble of clothing and mittens, often traded a dozen times a year. And at least occasionally, a fearsome itching follows this direct or indirect body contact. Tiny mites which burrow in the skin have passed from one person to another, and a great misery grips the victim.

You can usually identify scabies (the "seven-year itch") by spotting the burrows. Until scratch marks have confused the picture, these look like thin reddish streaks with tiny blisters at half-inch intervals or so all along them. They usually appear first on the arms, legs or body—practically never on the face—with the clincher (if present) being burrows on the webs between the fingers and along the sides of the digits.

Start your treatment with a prolonged hot bath and thorough soap-and-washcloth scrubbing. Follow immediately with a chin-to-toe application of 25 per cent benzyl benzoate emulsion or benzyl benzoate-DDT lotion, either obtainable at any drugstore. You'll usually need some help to be sure your whole back and other areas are covered. Repeat the application again the next morning BUT NOT ON ANY LATER OCCASION (extra repetitions often cause skin irritation and dermatitis). To avoid reinfection, check all other members of the family, and treat anyone with suspicious scratch marks or lesions simultaneously. Change to clean, hot-water laundered underwear and clothing, and either hot-water launder, dry clean or iron (ironing kills the mites, too) all clothes and bedclothes.

If itching continues after this treatment, it is usually due to skin irritation from the medicines and mildly infected scratch marks rather than from continued scabies. Starch or oatmeal baths (see above) generally give quick relief.

As an alternative program, slightly more expensive but much easier and less irritating to the skin, try Kwell cream or lotion. Bathe and dry thoroughly, then apply Kwell to all affected areas and do not wash off for 24 hours. One application usually does the trick.

Head lice, body lice, crab lice and bedbugs. Many years ago, my father (who was an eminent skin specialist) examined an obviously wealthy, superbly groomed woman who complained of an itching scalp. He could find nothing wrong, so he advised her to come back in a week without washing her hair. The cause of her misery literally galloped into view, and he exclaimed:

"Madam, you are lousy!"

Ignoring her stunned expression, he instructed that everyone in the household be treated at once, all the bedclothing boiled or ironed and so forth.

"But you don't understand," the patient said. "I have the most crucial house guests—how can I ever tell the central committee of the D.A.R. that they may all have head lice?"

I don't know whether anything helped this poor woman bear up under her social anguish, but it might give her some comfort to know that her story has relieved a great many people from any feeling of shame at encountering lice. It happens in the best of families, no matter how clean and careful you might be.

For either head lice or crab lice (found in pubic hair and armpits) Kwell shampoo is a definitely superior treatment. It kills both the lice and their nits (eggs which adhere to the hair). One thorough application usually suffices. DDT powder or lotion also kills the lice, but to avoid recurrence you usually have to trim the hair quite short and comb it very carefully with a fine-toothed metal comb to remove all nits. For body lice or "cooties" Kwell cream or lotion works very well. If you don't actually see the lice but get insect bites on exposed body areas, check carefully for bedbugs. Caladryl or other soothing treatment suffices for the bites, but you may need anything from DDT to a professional exterminator to rid yourself of the problem.

LEISURE TIME SKIN ASSAULTS

From the hordes of pallid Easterners who stream into Minnesota's wide open spaces every year, it seems safe to assume that almost everyone is spending more time outdoors these days. At times, traffic to the far wilderness is almost bumper to bumper around the Fourth of July. Along with the extra fun, more outdoor life brings miseries like insect bites, poison ivy rash and sunburn. Believe me, the Land of Lakes has given home remedies for these ailments a thorough trial!

Bee sting. If you get hives or severe general reaction to bee sting, you should check with your doctor for special medicine you can carry around with you. Such allergic reactions to bee sting sometimes become more and more severe until they become really serious or even fatal. Ordinary bee sting, which causes pain and swelling only in the vicinity of the sting itself, responds well to home measures.

Knifetip scraping. Most people make the mistake of trying to grasp the stinger with their fingers or with tweezers when they suffer a bee sting. In the process, they squeeze on the poison sac at the outer end of the stinger and make their ultimate reaction much worse. You should remove the stinger by gentle scraping with the tip of a sharp knife.

Ammonia solution. Ammonia helps to neutralize the formic acid which makes bee stings and ant bites painful. Mix two teaspoonfuls of household ammonia with one glass of water and use as a soak or compress immediately, before the sting opening has a chance to seal. Wasp and yellowjacket stings also respond to ammonia.

Nerve numbing agents. Ointments and lotions which make the pain nerves in the area insensitive definitely lessen the discomfort you suffer from a beesting. Surfacaine cream numbs surface nerves safely. The same pain relieving ingredient is combined with a preparation which fights later swelling in the very useful Surfadil lotion. Your druggist sells both preparations without requiring a prescription.

Mosquito and other insect bites. Itching insect bites respond best to soothing and antihistamine-containing lotions. Caladryl lotion works fairly well. Surfadil is very effective, too. If you do not have these on hand, a paste of bicarbonate of soda and water sometimes gives some comfort.

Poison ivy. The first time you get poison ivy, the rash usually develops 10 days or so after your exposure. Later attacks come on within a few hours. Ivy rash often spreads beyond the area of actual contact, but this spread results from the skin's sympathetic response to distant irritation instead of from contact with the blister fluid as many people think. You can break ivy blisters safely without spreading the irritation.

Unroofing blisters. You can usually make ivy dry up more quickly by taking the tops off of the blisters. Wipe the area with rubbing alcohol or clean it thoroughly beforehand. Use a flamed needle to open small blisters. Scissors and tweezers work best for taking the roofs off large fluid-filled pockets.

Soothing compresses. Mix two tablespoonfuls of Burow's solution, which you can get at any drug store without a prescription, with one glassful of lukewarm water. Wet cloths with this solution and apply to the itching areas. Cover with a layer of plastic sheeting or with a plastic refrigerator bag and leave in place for 30 to 45 minutes. Repeat four times daily.

Lotions. For milder forms of poison ivy or for healing cases, zinc oxide lotion is very soothing. For even faster results when the area involved is small, get your doctor to prescribe a fluorinated cortisone-type lotion, which usually dries up ivy in two to three days.

Sunburn. If you get a small patch of sunburn where your arm has hung out of the car window or where shirtsleeves have proved shorter than the ones you were accustomed to, Surfacaine cream will give you a lot of relief. For any substantial body area, however, Surfacaine cannot be used. These measures deserve a try:

Double strength Burow's. Two-thirds cupful of Burow's solution with enough water to make one pint is good for sunburn. If a wide area is involved, you may want to use tablets or powders to mix a larger quantity. Ask your druggist for directions. However you prepare the solution, wet several light towels, handkerchiefs, or strips of sheeting with it and apply to the burned area. In severe burns, you will probably want to use such applications for one hour out of each two, while milder burns may respond to 20 minute applications two or three times a day.

Calamine lotion. When you cannot use wet applications or for milder sunburn, try calamine lotion. However, be sure that you get plain rather than phenolated lotion, and buy a small bottle of glycerin to remove lotion crusts.

Ice for Sunburn. If you can freeze a sunburnt area just as the skin reaction is occurring, you can often cut down the damage quite substantially. The most dramatic demonstration of this I've seen occurred in my own family, where one of the youngsters was becalmed on a sunbathed lake at the very start of the season and reached shore just as her skin was starting to get red. We were camped far from any source of extra ice but used what we had on one side of her back. The other side blistered and became very sore, but the treated side hardly even got red. The technique is given in detail under "the instant freeze for burns" in the next chapter.

BLACKHEAD AND PIMPLE PROBLEMS

Don't treat all "zits" as acne. Raised reddish spots on the face and shoulders often come from dermatitis (see above), especially if the spots come up very quickly, are itchy instead of tender, and feel fairly pliable and soft. Dermatitis clears without being picked or squeezed and does not leave pits or scars. Mild acne may not drain or scar, but at least some of the pimples usually come to a head.

The outer layers of skin are made up of dead cell shells. Minor chemical changes, resulting at least partly from diet, can let those shells heap up around the openings of your skin's oil glands. This plugs the oil glands and causes blackheads, pimples or skin cysts. You can attack this chain of events at several points.

Diet. Whether or not you "are what you eat," your food choices have a lot to do with skin texture. Nuts and nut products, including peanut butter, and carbonated beverages seem to be the biggest factors in producing pimples. Although some recent studies seem to disagree, most of my patients also do better without chocolate and fried or fatty foods (including potato chips, french fries and fried-center hamburgers).

Vitamin A. Large quantities of Vitamin A help to condition your skin cells. The change increases oil gland openings and makes blackheads or pimples much less likely to appear. Use 50,000 unit tablets three times a day. Effects may be rather gradual, so it takes about a six-week trial to tell whether you are getting any help. There have been some reports that very prolonged (many years) use of this Vitamin can produce kidney stones, so check with your doctor before extending your treatment time beyond one year.

Skin-thinning soaps. Especially for acne on the shoulders and back, Lava soap or Mechanic's grit soap often works wonders. Rub the cake directly on the areas usually affected to thin the skin slightly and open up oil pores. Once a pimple has started this treatment does no good. Don't rub on the tender, raised pimples. Several showers a week with firm friction on the nontender affected areas will usually keep shoulder and back pimples under fairly good control.

Drying lotions. If you can shrink your skin slightly with a drying lotion, the pores and oil gland openings gape open. This prevents pimples and blackheads from getting a start. White lotion U.S.P. is the standard preparation, which any druggist can supply. Acnomel and several other trade preparations combine drying lotions with pimple-covering pigment.

Perhaps because of the cover-up feature, most people do not use these lotions correctly. The idea is to open up skin glands and keep pimples or blackheads from forming in the first place, not to treat already-formed pimples. You should therefore apply the lotion to the entire affected area (usually the face and base of the neck) rather than to the pimples and blackheads themselves. Wash the area thoroughly at bedtime, apply the lotion and leave it in place until morning, when you can wash it off again.

Blackhead squeezing. Get a blackhead squeezer for about 25 cents at the nearest drugstore. This has small, spoon-shaped portions at each end with a smooth-rimmed hole in the center. Wipe off the area with rubbing alcohol and allow to dry. Place either the larger or the smaller hole (whichever matches the size of the blackhead best) directly over the blackhead. Press the squeezer straight into the skin, without allowing to slide or skid along the skin at all. The contents of the blackhead should pop through the hole like a little white worm before the pressure reaches an uncomfortable level.

If a blackhead will not pop with the amount of pressure you can readily tolerate, you can soften its top with warm, wet cloths for ten minutes. Hot towels or "facial saunas" increase oil gland activity and make the underlying condition worse, though, so you should use them only when other methods fail.

Pimple picking. As long as a pimple is hard, you should never squeeze or pick it. The worst acne pustules and pitted scars result from squeezing a pimple before the skin covering has thinned out, so that the pus has no way to burst but inward. Most pimples will point up in a whitehead, with a thinned-out bit of transparent skin confining the drop of pus underneath. Some remain red in the center but become very soft and loose at the drainable spot. Until one or the other of these changes occurs, you should not pick or pinch at a pimple.

To open a pointed-up pimple, first pass the point of a needle through the flame of a match two or three times. Put the needle on the edge of your kitchen counter with the point hanging untouched in open air. Wipe off the pimple with rubbing alcohol. Hold the needle parallel with the skin and insert its point from the edge of the whitehead or central softness toward its center. Pull straight up away from the skin, breaking through a few skin cells. Press gently with a blackhead squeezer to see whether pus will break through, and if not pick slightly deeper. If you cause either oozing or flow of blood, stop and make gentle pressure through a cotton ball or gauze pad until the bleeding stops (usually three to four minutes without peeking). Do not squeeze pus through a bleeding surface—open blood vessels give the germs in pus a ready passage into your system, sometimes causing infection to spread.

Antibiotics and other prescription care. Very deep or painful pustules sometimes call for antibiotics. X-ray treatment or surface freezing may cause great improvement. Board-like or pitted skin can sometimes be thinned by surgical sandpapering. These measures are expensive and long drawn out, but they may be much better than the psychologic and social effects of permanently scarred and disfigured skin. Your family doctor should be able to give you some help with severe pimples, or to help you to locate a specialist who can give greater aid.

CHAPTER ELEVEN

Home Care for
Everyday Injuries

Here in Minnesota it's always open season for injuries. Skiing sprains, fishermen's falls, campers' ax cuts, and hunters' wounds keep the bandage business brisk. Home accidents which you might expect in any of the 50 states keep Minnesotans hopping, too. Bruises, strains and sprains, scrapes, cuts, and burns add up to a considerable burden of misery which well-chosen home measures can greatly relieve. Even the smallest scratch involves some risk of infection, too: home measures often ward off serious trouble by keeping wounds clean.

HOME REMEDIES FOR BRUISES, STRAINS, AND SPRAINS

You can keep down swelling, disability, and pain in bruises, strains, and sprains by taking proper home measures immediately after you get hurt. You can speed your recovery from such injuries with proper home care. You need no special equipment or expensive materials to accomplish these ends: you probably have everything you need in your home right now.

How to make sure that you don't have a fracture. Suppose that you fall or bump yourself or twist your ankle. Before you decide upon home measures, you want to be sure that you have no broken bones. Here are the usual rules of thumb:

1. Even slight tenderness over the small bones of the fingers, hands, wrist, toes, foot, ankle, and nose may mean fracture.

2. Even slight tenderness over a bone that has been wrenched instead of struck may mean fracture. Bony tenderness in a twisted ankle or wrist has to come from pulled ligaments or from wrenched-loose bone. Only X-rays can reliably distinguish.

3. Changes in body contour other than simple swelling at the site

of injury almost always mean fracture. Compare the injured extremity with its mate, especially with regard to bony knobs or prominences. Any difference between the two sides calls for a doctor's evaluation.

4. If jolting or compression conveyed along the shaft of the injured bone causes pain, fracture is almost always present. When you press straight back on your breastbone, for instance, rib fractures at the side of your chest usually hurt. Thumping on the bottom of the heel usually causes pain in any fracture from above the ankle to the hip. Thumping on the elbow or outstretched fist in such a way as to send a jolt straight up along the arm bones has similar effect. Naturally, you should use this maneuver only as a final check if no other evidence points strongly toward fracture.

5. *Any* pain in the middle of your back after a fall deserves a 'phone call to your doctor *before you attempt to get up.*

Two further cautions: Don't regard ability to move a part or put your weight on it as proof that the bones are intact. And don't assume that the part that hurts the worst is the one most seriously injured. If you have a serious fall or accident, run your hands over each extremity and each rib, check for tenderness in your abdomen and neck, and test for painless motion in each part of your spine before you try to get up.

How to hold down damage from a bruise, strain, or sprain. For the first 24 hours or more, the key remedies for any bruising or wrenching injury are cold applications, snug elastic bandages, gravity-aided blood drainage, and rest. Your aim at this stage is to prevent the leakage of fluid or blood from damaged blood vessels in the bruised or torn body parts. Cold shrinks those blood vessels, elastic bandages and gravity-aided blood drainage cut leakage from them, and rest lets them seal off leaks thoroughly and quickly. Here are specific techniques for applying these basic remedies:

Ice application. With ordinary bumps and bruises, you should apply ice immediately. Wrap an ice cube or a handful of crushed ice in a towel or washcloth and moisten the cloth with cold water. Apply directly to the injured area for ten to fifteen minutes. Do not put ice into direct contact with your skin, since it will sometimes cause a frost burn.

Ice bags. For sprained or strained ankles, large bruises, and other injuries to areas as large as the palm of your hand, you will probably find a padded ice bag the most convenient way to apply cold. An inexpensive plastic refrigerator bag works very well. Fill it about half way with crushed ice, add two or three tablespoonfuls of cold water, double or twist the open end and seal with a rubber band, and wrap the whole arrangement with a moist towel. Apply directly to the injured area for 10 to 15 minutes.

Cold clothes or soaks. If the injured area is larger than the palm of your hand or if you have no ice available, you may want to use cold cloths or soaks. Water fresh from the tap should be cold enough, even in areas where the pipes aren't as deeply buried as ours in the North Country. Soak the entire injured part for twenty to thirty minutes, adding fresh cold water or ice occasionally to keep the water cold. If you want to use cold cloths, fold a towel over until it is six or eight layers thick, dip it in cold water, wring it partially dry and apply to the injured part. Change as often as necessary to keep it cold. Continue for half an hour.

Elastic bandages. You can often keep down swelling in an injured extremity by putting on an elastic bandage. The rubber-containing brands work best. Wind the bandage in a spiral with about half its width overlapping on each turn. It should be snug, not too tight: if you apply it stretched about half as far as possible, you will find it just snug enough. When you have finished with your elastic bandage, wash it in lukewarm water with mild soap and dry it by draping it in loops along a line, so that the whole weight of the bandage does not stretch one end of it out of shape.

Gravity-aided blood drainage. If blood goes definitely downhill in the veins which lead from an injured area to the heart, injured vessels have less pressure and congestion in them. This reduces seepage of fluid and blood.

You can provide this kind of gravity-aided drainage in several ways. With bruises, strains and sprains of the hand or wrist, a properly adjusted sling will hold your hand at shoulder height in the daytime. When you lie down, let your hand rest on your chest and adjust a couple of pillows under your elbow and upper arm. You can improve drainage from a hurt foot or ankle by placing two pillows under the lower leg. Keep the lower leg level with the floor, since tight leaders in the back of the knee block circulation slightly if the leg is propped up straight.

Rest. Almost every athlete I know thinks that he can cut down trouble from a bruise or sprain if he works the injured part right away. Unfortunately, just the opposite is true: exercise makes any bruising or rending injury worse until swelling has reached its peak and started to subside, which usually takes about 24 hours. You can use splinting or adhesive strapping according to the techniques described in the next section as soon as you can get the necessary equipment together. Meanwhile, don't use the affected part any more than you can help.

How to speed recovery from a bruise, strain, or sprain. After swelling has reached its peak and started to subside, you need home remedies to help speed your body's processes of repair. You want to draw more circulating blood to the area, break up congestion and hold torn tissues steady in their proper places while they mend. Here are several effective techniques:

Heat. After swelling reaches its peak, which usually takes about 24 hours, heat helps more than cold. At this stage, you want to open up nearby blood vessels so that they can carry away the fluid and blood which leaked from the injured (but now sealed) vessels. Hot soaks or hot wet towels for 30 minutes three or four times a day benefit any bruise, strain, or sprain. As you add hot water or re-dip your towels, always check the temperature with your uninjured hand: otherwise, the treated part may become sufficiently accustomed to heat to let you burn yourself. A good many of our Minnesota housewives can be even more precise: after years of seeing how ladies with candy thermometers win more prizes at the state and county fairs, they've stormed the hardware stores for such equipment. Comes time for hot applications and they can keep the water at exactly 112 degrees, which is perfect!

Massage. One thing you have to give our farm families: each member will do almost anything for the others. Whenever anybody gets a bruise, strain, or sprain, they'll all pitch in to help heal it up faster. Massage definitely improves circulation and speeds healing with all these problems. Here's the exact technique for bruises or strains of the leg:

> Lie down with the injured part bared and arranged comfortably on two or more pillows. Have your helper powder the leg thoroughly from ankle to thigh with talc or bath powder. He should rub gently with the palm of the hand and with limp fingers, starting from midcalf level and stroking up toward the hip. Strokes should be gentle, rhythmic, and all in the same direction. Your helper should gradually increase the pressure applied at the center of each stroke, but should begin and end each stroke gently and smoothly throughout the treatment. Your helper can make his strokes as if your leg were a piece of clay he is shaping into a gracefully tapered vase. Massage should move closer and closer to the swollen, tender area, but should never quite reach it: your object is to improve circulation in the part, not to rub or work the injured area. Twenty minutes of stroking once a day usually speeds healing quite substantially.

Similar massage works well for injuries of the arm.

Strapping. You can brace most strained or sprained joints very effectively with adhesive strapping. If you have to put tape on a very hairy part, dry-shave the area first with a safety razor and a new blade. You will usually find that tape goes on best if you cut an approximate length and apply the middle first, allowing both ends to seek the exact sites at which they lie down most smoothly. Tape should always be laid on instead of put on under tension. If you want to pull a part in a given direction with tape, turn it that way and apply the tape without further pull. If tape tends to irritate your skin somewhat, apply a coat of tincture of benzoin and let it dry before putting on the adhesive. You can always make narrower strips from whatever width tape you have on hand by cutting a length, nicking the end, and tearing lengthwise. Here are the exact techniques you should use to strap each of the most common strains and sprains:

Stubbed small toe. All the toes except the big toe work together as a unit when you walk. If one of them gets hurt, you can make it much more comfortable by strapping the four smaller toes together. Cut four foot-long strips of half-inch adhesive tape. With the toes relaxed and in their natural position, slip the center of one strip between the big toe and its neighbor, with its sticky side toward the smaller toes, as close to the base of the toe as possible. Lay the upper end of the tape across the top of the toes, and smooth its loose end down along the side of your little toe and the sole of your foot. Lay the bottom end of the tape along the bottom of the toes so that it crosses the upper strip on the outer side of the little toe and ends on the top of your foot. Slip another strip of tape between the big toe and its neighbor. Overlap about half its width and run it parallel to the first strip. Continue in this fashion until all four strips have been applied. The last two or three strips will tend to cross at the ends of the toes instead of at the outer side of the foot, but this will remain comfortable so long as the tape is laid on instead of pulled tight.

Sprained big toe. You can strap your big toe all by itself. Cut three strips of half-inch tape each eight inches long. With the toe straight and relaxed, stick the middle of one strip fairly low down on the end of the toe. Direct the ends so that they will cross above the far toe joint and run up along the top of the foot. Apply the other strips back along the toe overlapping half their width, then gently lay two or three circular turns of tape around the toe itself.

Arch strain. Pain on the outer side of the foot after a wrenching injury usually comes from an arch strain. You can speed healing by taking the stretch off the injured ligaments and bracing them. One-inch adhesive works best. Cut three strips of tape about one foot long. Turn the foot and heel inward. Apply the middle of one adhesive strip diagonally across the outer side of the heel and bring the ends around so that one crosses the inner side of the foot just below the ankle bone and the other comes up over the arch. Apply the other two strips similarly, overlapping about half their width. Now cut three slightly longer strips of tape. Turn the front part of the foot outward as far as it will go. Apply the center of one adhesive strip to the sole of the foot just behind the base of your toes. Lead both ends up across the top of the foot and back around the arch. Apply the other two strips approximately parallel, overlapping about half their width at the start. Now apply circular strips of tape over the rest of the arch to make the whole dressing into a smooth, foot-covering sheet.

Strained or sprained ankle. So long as the most tender spot in a turned ankle is *below* instead of *at* the tip of the ankle bone, you probably have a sprain or strain instead of a fracture. Use three strips of one inch adhesive tape each about thirty inches long and a three inch elastic bandage for a satisfactory home dressing. Turn the foot sharply outward on the ankle. Apply the middle of one strip of tape across the bottom of the heel so that the ends lead up both sides of the ankle. If the shape of your leg does not permit a symmetrical, stirrup-like strapping, be sure that the end going up the outer side of your leg goes straight up even if the other end tends to wind toward the front of the leg or around the foot. Apply the other two strips of tape more or less parallel and overlapping at the heel, and let their ends seek positions in which the tape lies down smoothly. Wrap the elastic bandage on top of the tape, starting with an anchor turn around the ankle, then taking alternate turns around the ankle and the arch, and then spiraling up the leg.

Strained or sprained thumb. When an accident bends your thumb back, the joint at its base usually gives. Hold this joint straight while you strap it. First put two strips of half inch tape lengthwise along the top of the thumb from tip to wrist. Cut five strips of half inch tape about one foot long. Place the middle of one strip across the palmar portion of the tip of the thumb. Direct the ends so that they will spiral up the thumb onto the back and the heel of the hand. Place further parallel strips overlapping up the thumb until the entire thumb is covered and the fan of tape from its base spreads to about half of the wrist. Two or three circular turns of adhesive around the wrist help to anchor the tape ends so that they will not curl up and come loose.

Strained or sprained finger. You can strap a mildly sprained finger with adhesive with the method just described by spiraling up from the tip and fanning out along the back of the hand. One or two strips of tape around the hand at the base of the fingers will anchor the tape ends.

Baseball fingers. For severely sprained fingers or fingers injured by a blow into the fingertip, the hairpin splint makes a very effective and comfortable dressing. You need a little flexible collodion (which you can buy without a prescription), some gauze roller bandage (preferably one inch wide), and one or two old fashioned U-shaped hairpins. Wind two layers of bandage on the finger as smoothly as possible. With a small pledget of cotton or an applicator stick, wet the bandage with collodion and allow to dry for two or three minutes. Shape the hairpin to the upper surface of the finger and hold it in place with two more layers of gauze. Moisten with collodion again. If you are planning to work with the injured hand, shape another hairpin to the front of the finger. Apply two more layers of gauze and wet with collodion. Apply more gauze and collodion until you have built a sturdy dressing, allowing each layer to dry thoroughly before applying the next. If you have trouble with the gauze coming loose, wind it diagonally in such a way that both ends are up on the palm of the hand where you can hold them until the collodion sets, then trim them off.

Strained or sprained wrist. You can strap a sprained wrist fairly effectively with the hand in the tipped-up position. First apply a strip of two inch adhesive along the top of the tipped-up wrist from the knuckles to the middle of the forearm. Cut three strips of one inch adhesive about two feet long. Apply the middle of one strip across the palm of the hand at the base of the fingers. Direct the ends so that they cross at the middle of the back of your hand and again in front of the wrist. Apply further strips with considerable overlap on the palm of the hand, but direct the ends to make the overlap decrease somewhat along the course of the tape. A two-inch elastic bandage gives an ideal finish to the dressing. Wind it around the wrist first, wind two or three turns alternately around the wrist and the hand, then spiral up the forearm. If an elastic bandage is not available, finish the dressing with two or three circular turns of tape around the midforearm.

Persistent discomfort in sprains or strains. An injured ligament should heal in ten to fourteen days. If discomfort continues after this time, strapping seldom does any good. At this point, you should switch to contrast baths. Bathe the whole part, not just the sore place. Soak the affected part in warm water (105° F.) for four minutes, in cold water (50° F.) for one minute, then back into the warm Continue alternating, four minutes warm and one minute cold, for about 30 minutes. Always begin and end with warm.

Massage, as described above, is especially effective if performed immediately after a contrast bath.

Blown-up knee or elbow bursa. After unaccustomed activity or injury, you might abruptly develop a painful swelling at the front of your knee or above the point of your elbow. This generally comes from bleeding into a bursa, which is a smooth-walled collapsed sack (like an empty balloon with a few drops of oil in it). Bursas normally occur at friction points between muscle and tendon layers and act as bearings when adjacent structures rub against one another. If injury or strain breaks a tiny blood vessel inside a bursa, there is no pressure to help stop the bleeding until the entire bursa has filled. By that time, enough blood is in the space to keep the area sore for two or three weeks.

Treatment for this condition is just like that described for bruises, but is somewhat more urgent. If you can chill the part right away, before much bleeding has occurred, you may stop hemorrhage immediately. A firm pressure dressing also helps, with a three-inch elastic bandage for the elbow or a four-inch one for the knee. Apply this in figure-eight style, with one loop above the joint and one below (crossing in the fold, not over the swollen bursa). By working up and down, you can cover the affected area with a firm, well-anchored bandage which will not separate at the crucial area when the extremity is bent, as a spiral bandage does.

Best continue cold applications two or three times a day and pressure bandages between for three days or so. Lukewarm soaks can be substituted for the cold applications thereafter, to speed absorption of the blood and aid healing.

Other bruising or wrenching injuries. Special home measures are very helpful for smashed fingers or toes, sprained knees, and sprained backs. Here's what to do about these common problems:

Mashed fingers or toes. A mashed finger or toe often shows a blue-black puddle of blood underneath the nail. This form of bruising causes severe discomfort because the accumulated blood presses on highly sensitive nerve endings. It also leads to loss of the nail unless the pressure is promptly relieved. First step is thorough cleanliness: wash your hands well and wipe off the affected finger with rubbing alcohol so that you will not get germs into the space underneath the nail while draining the blood out. Then follow one of these three methods:

Hot paper clip drainage. Unwind the first two turns of a metal paper clip and heat the free end to white heat with a cigarette lighter, gas flame or candle. Steady the injured finger against the tabletop and touch the hot paper clip end to the center of the blue-black area. If the blackish blood does not drain out, reheat the metal and apply it again until you burn a hole all the way through the nail (about 1/16 of an inch).

Knifetip drilling. Clean a sharp, pointed penknife blade and the injured finger thoroughly with rubbing alcohol. Steady the injured finger against a tabletop, and press the point of the knife gently into the center of the blue-black area. Twist the knifeblade clockwise and counterclockwise for ninety degrees or more, gradually increasing pressure. When you have drilled through the nail, blackish blood will ooze out of the first needlepoint-sized hole. Wipe away the blood with a freshly ironed handkerchief or sterile pad, and pick away at the margins of the hole with the knife point until it is as large as the eye in a small needle.

Nail margin peeling. A badly mashed finger may reaccumulate blood after the hole you burn or drill has sealed off. If so, the blood often works its way to the edge of the nail. Whenever there is a blue-black margin of skin at the edge of the nail, you will find that the easiest and most comfortable way to drain the puddled blood away is by peeling the discolored skin away from the nail edge with a blunt nail file. If the blood does not drain out during the peeling process, you will find that the skin layer inside the blue-black margin is dead like the top of a blister, and can be pierced and torn back with a flamed needle or gently opened with the corner of a new razorblade.

After-care. As long as blood seeps from a hole in or around the nail, keep a clean, dry bandage in place. If the nail begins to separate, trim the loose margins short with clippers so that they will not catch and tear the rest of the nail loose. As the new nail grows in, it will push the old one loose without pain or danger.

Sprained knees. As long as a sprained knee is sore and swollen, your best bet is to use cold compresses, hot towels, rest, and elastic bandaging. Cold helps most during the first 24 hours, as often as you can get around to it (but not more than one hour out of every two). Hot wet towels thereafter for half an hour three or four times a day often help. A severely sprained knee should keep you off your foot for several days either on crutches or strictly at home with only such walking as is necessary for self-care. A three- or four-inch elastic bandage helps a lot. Wrap the knee partially bent. Anchor the bandage with one or two turns below the knee, then run diagonally up the back of the knee, around the thigh and diagonally down the back of the knee. Use this above-and-below winding as you overlap each turn perhaps half the bandage width until the joint is firmly braced.

Healing sprains and trick knees. If your knees sometimes lock or give way, torn ligaments or cartilages are usually at fault. Even mild sprains leave ligaments weak and relaxed. In either case, you need to build knee bracing muscle strength. Certain of your thigh muscles bridge the knee with what can become a sturdy, bracing girdle of muscle fibers. You can keep your knee completely stable even if one of its ligaments is completely torn away, by building tone in these muscles. Do this exercise three times a day for three weeks, and once daily thereafter:

> Sit in a straight chair with your leg stretched out straight in front of you. Set the muscles at the front of your thigh hard, pulling the kneecap up toward your hip, for five seconds. Keeping the muscle firm, slowly raise your heel about four inches off the floor. Hold the leg in this position for about five seconds. Let the heel down slowly, keeping the thigh muscles set. Relax the thigh muscle after another five seconds. After a five second rest, repeat. Continue for five to ten contractions.

How to cure back sprains and strains. Better than 9 out of 10 patients with low back strain severe enough to drive them to hospital care got complete relief with a program of rest, exercise, and postural training which you can closely mimic in your own home. Here are the five steps which many of my patients have used in their own homes to move from back misery to permanent relief.

1. Rest in the jackknife position. Buy a piece of one inch plywood to fit between your coil or box springs and your mattress. If you have an innerspring mattress, place the plywood on top of it and obtain a cotton mattress to place on that. Saw across the plywood (or ask the lumberyard man to do so) about 30 inches from the top, and install hinges. Run one thickness of masking tape or cloth tape around the edges to avoid splinters in your fingers while making the bed. Raise the head end of the board to a 45-degree angle and prop up your knees with a blanket roll or two pillows. Although this position seems uncomfortable at first, it often gives prompt

relief. Later, you will want to use the same bedding in the flat position for several months or years during recovery.

For the first 24 to 48 hours of treatment, you must stay in bed continuously, use a bed pan as necessary, and eat your meals in bed. Use extreme care never to stretch or stiffen the back. Let your body weight press into the jackknife angle to ease tightness in your back muscles.

2. Learn to keep the lower back flat while carrying on normal activities by taking a series of exercises in bed. Start by lying on your back with your knees bent and your feet flat on the bed. Roll the pelvis forward, as if you were a burlesque artist doing a bump. Hold it for three to five seconds, with the muscles of your abdomen and buttocks tense and hard. Relax for several seconds and repeat 5 to 10 times. Then draw up one knee toward your armpit, pulling with both hands. Draw up the other knee, stretching the back muscles thoroughly. Repeat the whole procedure several times a day. After you have mastered this back-flattening technique of tilting your pelvis, try to keep your pelvis tipped and your lower back flat as you straighten one leg at a time and then as you raise your head and shoulders.

3. Learn to get out of bed, stand, and move about without ever letting a hollow appear in your lower back. Keep one knee clutched against your chest while you are getting your other foot on the ground at first, until you learn to get up without letting your back arch backward. Use the wall as a guide while you learn to stand and move. Stand with your feet four to six inches away from the wall and your back flattened against it. Keep your spine flat against the wall as you raise first one leg, then the other. Squat down and stand back up again without letting your spinal curve change. Keep the spinal curve unchanged as you shift your weight onto your toes and rock away from the wall, then back to it. Finally, walk away from the wall with your lower back completely flat and your pelvis tipped forward instead of back.

4. Learn to perform even extreme bodily movements without letting a hollow form over your lower spine. Lie on your back with your knees bent and your feet flat on the bed, keep your back flattened and touch your toes with your fingertips. Keep your back flat as you squat down on your heels and return to the standing position.

5. Drill yourself in assuming all the positions and carrying out all the motions which your job requires without ever letting a hollow form in the small of your back.

This program for curing back injuries works. Take aspirin four times a day after each meal and at bedtime to keep comfortable while you apply rest, exercise, and retraining: two tablets at a dose if you weigh less than 150 pounds, three to a dose if you weigh more. Check Chapter One for further measures you can apply for any nagging, persistent back discomfort.

How to prevent recurrent back injuries. Your back ligaments never heal quite as strong as they started. If you once injure your back, you can often save yourself a lot of misery by watching your footing, keeping your back upright while you lift, and by lifting with your legs instead of your back.

When your doctor can give worthwhile aid with backache and back injury. Your doctor can always give worthwhile aid with these three kinds of back trouble:

1. Back pain without strain, injury, or overuse often stems from disease of the kidneys, reproductive organs, spinal column or other vital body parts. Your doctor can identify the source of such trouble, and usually can give quick, permanent relief.

2. Back pain following a severe fall or injury deserves a doctor's care on the spot. If a bone is broken in the spine, there is definite risk of lifelong damage to the spinal cord even if pain is not severe. Your doctor can keep that risk under control.

3. Any back trouble that persists in spite of home measures or requires strong, prescription-only medicines for its relief deserves a doctor's care. In most such cases, your doctor can bring relief with a more intense program based on the same principles outlined above. In a few cases, special braces, injections, or surgery may prove to be the quickest means of getting well.

HOW TO HEAL CUTS, SCRAPES, AND BURNS

You can heal most minor injuries with simple home measures. Four key steps are:

1. Clean the wound.
2. Keep germs from getting in.
3. Improve circulation.
4. Bandage or splint to assure rest and protection as the wound heals.

How to tell when you can get worthwhile help from a doctor for cuts, scrapes or burns. Your doctor can speed healing of most cuts, scrapes, and burns.

A cut that goes all the way through the skin heals more quickly if it is pulled together, either with tape or with stitches. You can tell whether the cut is deep enough to need such care by moving one edge in and out or back and forth. If you can move one edge more than an eighth of an inch without the other edge moving, your doctor can help you with stitches or taping.

Scraped places may have ground-in dirt that you can't scrub loose without undue pain. If so, see your doctor. Be sure your lockjaw protection is up to date if you are hurt in any area to which animal wastes may have been tracked or if you cannot wash to the very bottom of the wound.

A burn that turns dead-white or scorched in the center deserves a doctor's care no matter how small it is. Large blistering burns benefit by measures you can't easily apply at home.

Your doctor has tremendous weapons against infection nowadays. Redness, swelling, red streaks up your arm or leg, sore kernels in your neck, armpit or groin, throbbing pain, fever, or chills call for germ-killing medicines, which will work much more quickly if you let your doctor put them to work for you right away.

How to clean out a cut or scrape. The first thing to do for a cut or scrape is to wash with soap and water. Clean your hands thoroughly as you start—hands normally have more germs than any other surface part of your body. Then wash the wound, using either gauze pads or clean, ironed handkerchiefs as washcloths. Soap the cloth and wash with gentle rubbing while the sore is actually in a soft stream of water from a spigot or pitcher. Use at least one quart of water for each wound.

Soap and water actually prevent five times as many infections as any antiseptic used in the depths of a wound. Antiseptics used in a scrape or cut kill tiny portions of the tender tissue underneath your skin. This leaves dead material as food for any remaining germs, and actually does harm instead of good.

How to use antiseptics. The next thing to do is put an antiseptic paint like mercurochrome, merthiolate or metaphen on the normal skin around your sore. Germs always can be found inside the sweat glands, even on freshly washed skin. If you do nothing about these germs, they work back to the surface, rub along the inside of the bandage, and get into your wound within twenty minutes. Antiseptic on the unbroken skin cuts down the number of germs that get into the sore without doing any damage to living tissue. Use antiseptics, but use them *around* a wound instead of *inside* it.

How to improve circulation in the healing sore. Better circulation gives better ability to fight germs and quicker healing. Gentle pressure of an elastic bandage applied smoothly from foot to knee helps leg wounds by keeping down swelling and congestion. Propping an injured leg above breast level also helps. On the hand or arm, you usually need a sling to keep the hurt part up, so that blood runs downhill to the heart. You can rig a sling out of a square yard of muslin or sheeting. Fold the square diagonally to make a triangular bandage. Tie the two sharp corners together at the back of the neck with the wrist resting on the middle of the fold and the bandage's blunt angle at the elbow. Adjust so that the lower arm is comfortably raised. Pull the excess cloth back until the sling is smooth from wrist to elbow, fold this excess around the elbow and pin it to the inside surface of the sling.

How to bandage a cut or scrape. The final thing to do for a sore is treat it gently and protect it as it heals. If injured tissue from beneath the skin or healing tissue is exposed, put some petroleum jelly or mild antiseptic ointment on the inside of the bandages or use bandages with plastic lined pads (Telfa) to avoid sticking. If you get hurt on your hands or arms, make your bandage six or eight layers thick to brace the parts and keep them from moving too much. I remember one patient who had a small cut on his finger, for instance.

"I've been fooling with this for a week," he said to me. "It just won't heal."

The cut was shallow and short, but it ran along the side of one finger joint. Whenever he bent his finger, the wound gaped open. His body couldn't build healing tissue fast enough on such shifting ground. A bulky bandage, in this case stiffened with a few matchstick-sized bits of wood, allowed his cut to mend in two days.

The instant freeze for burns. The most dramatically helpful home measure added in this edition is undoubtedly the instant freeze for burns. I've seen dozens of injuries which would have gone on to blister formation or worse stopped almost instantly by immediate cold applications. Not only does this program give prompt pain relief, it also cuts down on tissue damage and may prevent weeks of misery.

You need take no precautions against ice burns from overchilling, as described for other forms of cold application. Just get maximum cold to the spot as quickly as possible. Instant application of ice or snow is ideal. If large areas are burned, ice water soaks or compresses may spread the effect to make maximum use of available ice. If ice or snow are not available, perhaps you can get ice-cold water from a drinking fountain, or run the tap water until it is extremely cold. Whatever means you use, try to chill the part as much as possible and keep it chilled for at least fifteen minutes. Pain usually will disappear almost instantly with adequate chilling. Return of pain is a good guide to need for further cold applications. With severe burns, pain may return as soon as the part warms up, and cold applications must be replaced within five or ten minutes. With milder burns, discomfort only gradually reasserts itself, and applications for fifteen minutes every hour for two or three hours suffices. Generally speaking, any burn which requires constant chilling for more than one hour involves enough tissue damage to make a physician's care worthwhile. Danger of shock or other complications makes medical attention worthwhile with any burn covering more than ten per cent of the body surface.

Immediate chilling helps so much with burns that I would give it priority even over cleanliness. Even if you have to fish the ice out of someone's water glass or scoop up dirty snow from the side of the road, chill that burn instantly! You'll be amazed at the results.

Flame burns. If you burn yourself in a direct flame, the heat usually kills any germs present. Even though the wound looks grimy from soot, you can treat it as being already cleaned. Reddened areas without change in skin texture respond to greasy ointments like Burn Ointment U.S.P., which you can buy at any drugstore without a prescription. Blistered or scorched areas call for bandaging with petroleum jelly or Telfa. If you are going to see your doctor, cover the burn with a sterile gauze pad or with a freshly ironed handkerchief rather than use grease.

Scalds and other non-flame burns. Wash with soap and water and bandage exactly like a scrape or cut. Several layers of gauze or of fluffed handkerchiefs followed by a snug elastic bandage help to make smooth, even pressure. If blisters become as large as a quarter, you can speed healing by cutting off the dead skin roof. Use manicure scissors which have been flamed or soaked in alcohol, and similarly sterilized tweezers. Keep the scissors blades parallel to the skin and nick the edge of the blister. Insert one scissors blade in the nick and cut around the blister top near its edge, steadying the freed tissue with your tweezers. Discard the blister roof and bandage with petroleum-jelly-coated gauze or Telfa, several gauze pads and a snug gauze or elastic bandage.

Frostbite. Before I moved to Minnesota, the words "biting cold" didn't really mean anything to me. Cold was a penetrating, dank discomfort that went on to make you shiver with chill, not a painful pincer on exposed fingers, nose and ears. Here one almost welcomes painful blasts of wind—frostbite starts with numbness, so you begin to worry when discomfort ends! But cold injury in one form or another can occur anywhere, even in the balmiest climates, and folks all over the world could benefit from experience at Frostbite Falls.

Prevention still helps more than any cure. A lot of cold injury comes from exposure *below freezing* to parts chilled by damp clothing or immersion in slightly too-cold water. I've seen "trench foot" in spring and fall canoe campers who wore wet tennis shoes through a cold snap, for instance. Other cases stem from tight, binding clothes which both carry cold through at the creases and cut down circulation in the part. We've had a rash of frost injury lately due to snow-mobiling in ordinary winter clothes—the extra air movement as you swish around at forty miles an hour can nip an exposed finger or ear in a hurry.

Emergency treatment can make a tremendous difference when numbness, color change or loss of feeling makes you suspect cold injury. Most injury seems to occur through cold-induced spasm of blood vessels rather than tissue freezing itself. Warm soaks or compresses are the best way to open up those blood vessels again. However, if you apply heat directly to the affected part, warmth increases tissue need for fuel even faster than it increases circulation, and can occasionally cause both pain and further damage. You can get full benefit from warm applications by applying the warm compress to the affected body part (arm, leg, etc.) above the site of injury rather than to the injured zone itself. For a frostbitten hand, soak or compress the whole arm from the wrist up rather than from the wrist down, for instance—you'll open the blood vessels in the affected area without increasing tissue oxygen need. The hand itself can be loosely surrounded with flannel or wool to help hold warmth as the increased blood flow brings it, but should not be included in the soak or compress.

There are some body parts where this approach is not practical, of course. You can't soak your head for a frostbitten ear, and frostbite sometimes occurs on the torso where clothing creases or gapes. In these areas, direct thawing works best.

In either case, the water temperature should be 105 degrees, preferably measured with a candy or bath thermometer. Immersing an air thermometer will work, but usually the glass is so thick that temperature readings are not accurate for five minutes or so. If you do not have a thermometer, make the water lukewarm rather than hot—105 is considerably below the top temperature a healthy skin can stand (112 to 120 degrees depending on past dishwashing and similar exposure). *Never thaw a part which might become frozen again* before final treatment—this step makes gangrene and loss of tissue almost inevitable.

Any frostbite or cold injury which goes on to form blisters or in which sense of touch does not come back deserves a doctor's care. Cold injuries are notorious for seeming mild when later developments prove that they were serious. Above all, don't break blisters or apply any ointment, jelly or poultice—if the injury seems to require these measures, the possibility of lasting damage always justifies professional care.

Splinters. You can remove most splinters for yourself with a flamed needle and a pair of tweezers. Two key points: always unroof a splinter as far as possible before you try to move it, and always tease the splinter loose with the needle point before you try to pick it out with the tweezers. Here's the step-by-step technique:

> Clean the area thoroughly with rubbing alcohol. Pass the point of your needle through a flame several times. Slide the tip of the needle a hair's breadth into the hole along the splinter's upper surface. Turn the needle shaft down until it is parallel with the skin and lift up on its point, pulling loose a flake of dead surface skin. Repeat until one eighth of an inch or more of the splinter has been unroofed. Hook the tip of the needle underneath the exposed base of the splinter and gently test to see whether you can lift it. If so, move the splinter up and down and from side to side a couple of times. Transfer the needle to your left hand, and take the tweezers in your right hand. Lift up the splinter end with the point of the needle so that you can grasp it firmly with the tweezers, and remove it. Usually no bandage is necessary.

Splinters under a fingernail. You can cut a wedge of nail off of the top of a splinter and lift it free much more easily than you can pull it out the way it went in. Soak the finger in warm water for twenty minutes to soften the nail. Wipe it off with rubbing alcohol. Use the corner of an alcohol-soaked, clean razor blade. Start over the point of the splinter and make a shallow cut toward the end of the finger along one side of the splinter's shaft. Go back to the point of the splinter, and make another shallow cut toward the end of the finger in such a way that a small pie-shaped wedge of nail is defined over the splinter. Go over these shallow cuts several times, deepening them evenly. You will have to lighten your pressure as you approach the nail margin to keep from cutting yourself as the razor slips off the nail. When the cuts in the nail seem to be nearly or completely through, snip these neglected parts at the margin with scissors and peel the wedge back toward its point. Lift the splinter free with a needle point and pick it out. The wedge defect in the nail will disappear as the nail grows out.

Gouged out wounds. If you tear or cut out a bit of skin, the resulting wound is often quite painful. Small gouges will heal up with simple home measures, though. Put an old, freshly ironed handkerchief in a small covered oven dish with about an ounce of petroleum jelly. Heat in the oven until the petroleum jelly melts and soaks into the cloth. Let cool. Cut a piece of this material large enough to fold into three or four layers over the wound. Cover with a gauze and adhesive bandage. Change the bandage once a day. If the wound heals normally, pinkish proud flesh will form in two or three days, then grayish skin cells will make a pearly, glistening margin that gradually closes the defect. If the proud flesh heaps up so that the skin cells have to grow uphill, let your doctor burn them down with special chemicals. As soon as the whole wound has grayish, glistening tissue across it, you can omit further bandaging. A little cold cream rubbed into the area once or twice a day helps to keep the tender healing tissue from cracking open again.

CHAPTER TWELVE

Tonics and Correctives That Build Your Strength and Energy

As you drive through northern Minnesota, you will often notice a small windowless concrete hut nestled close to the shore of some river or lake. Don't make the mistake of calling the blond giants in the vicinity Swedes! They're almost certainly Finnish in descent, and quite proud of it. The concrete huts prove their dedication to a tone-up ritual originating in the Old Country, and unexcelled anywhere in the world—the famous "sauna." By pouring water on hot rocks, participants fill the little huts with thick, hot steam. The novices lie near the floor, while old hands rest on shelves closer to the ceiling where the rising heat may reach 140° F. The thick, moist warmth increases circulation in their naked skin until it looks quite flushed. Brisk flailing with wooden switches brings still more blood to the surface, whereupon the order of the day becomes a plunge in icy water. Surprisingly, the cold fluid feels like warm syrup to the still hot hide. When it begins to chill, a brisk toweling and warm clothes are close at hand. If you want a new sensation of vigor and vitality, any Finn will tell you that a sauna never fails!

We'll say more about home saunas later in this chapter, but most people must resort to less vigorous tonic methods for lack of equipment, companions, or courage. If you find weariness draining away the pleasures of life and keeping you from doing your best, if you find modern racecourse living imposing intolerable burdens of nervous and physical fatigue, if you suffer fatigue-inducing disorders or distress—you can certainly benefit from tonic techniques that build strength, zest, and energy. The tried-and-true methods described in this chapter help to combat everyday weariness and irritability, improve your mood and resistance, and nullify conditions which drag you down. Detailed directions will help you to fight five common disorders which increase fatigue, and to get effective help for several others.

HOW TO FIGHT TENSION AND FATIGUE WITH LIFE'S GREAT NATURAL TONICS

Perfectly normal, healthy people often need a soothing, reviving tonic technique. Tension builds up, irritability and restlessness cause distress, and blue moods or living reverses take their toll. Even for everyday vicissitudes, home tonic procedures are worthwhile. For paralyzing tension or depression, they help even more.

Part by part relaxation. The most important single way to conserve your energy is to dissolve excess tension with deliberate relaxation. When you are tense, every muscle in your body is working. You use just as much physical energy as if you were walking continuously at a rapid clip. No wonder you feel exhausted by the end of the day!

You can control tension and intensify the benefits of rest through the technique of part by part relaxation. Ordinary rest or simple relaxation leaves muscles in their basic state of tension. Deliberate, part-by-part relaxation goes beyond this point to deliberately probed depths of laxity. Here is the basic method:

> Lie on your back in a quiet room with your arms at your sides and your legs uncrossed. Deliberately relax your scalp muscles, your face muscles, then your neck. (If you have difficulty getting the muscles to relax at first, learn to relax by exaggerating muscle stiffness, then eliminating it. Hold your neck stiffer and stiffer by stages until it is extremely stiff. Then hold it not quite so stiff, still looser, and looser still. When you get back to normal tension, continue the same process by which you have moved from stiff to normal, and move on from normal to relaxed.) When your scalp, face, and neck seem fairly relaxed, move on to other parts of the body. Relax your right arm and hand, then your right leg, left leg, and left arm. Next, stretch your breathing muscles. Slowly take a deep breath through your nose, inflating your lungs as far as possible with your diaphragm, then further with the chest muscles. Let the breath escape gently through your mouth. Repeat the breathing exercise three times. Start with the scalp again, and impose even more complete relaxation on each of your body parts.

Part-by-part relaxation is fundamental to three tonic techniques. The first, most universally applicable, and easiest to learn, is the *rest break with part-by-part relaxation.* A rest break during the day with part-by-part relaxation is three to six times as effective as the same amount of extra rest at night. Most workers find the twenty minutes or half hour before supper an ideal time for a rest break, while housewives more commonly take their time off after lunch. The room should be darkened and quiet if possible. If physical weariness plagues you, extra benefit stems from propping your legs and arms on pillows. The knees should be slightly bent with the lower legs parallel to the floor on two pillows each. Turn your hands palm down on one pillow each with your arms slightly out from your sides. A very small pillow or rolled towel under the neck usually works better than a big, soft pillow. Follow the basic method for part-by-part relaxation described above.

Rest periods can do a lot for you, as Herman Saunders found out shortly after he was promoted to service manager at a large automobile agency.

"I'm racking myself up at work," he told me. "Between being on my feet all the time and constant pressure, I'm so tired and tense that I'm not worth a hang by afternoon."

There was nothing wrong with Herman except the natural effects of new responsibility and a heavy work load. A noon hour rest break helped a lot. He took a full hour lunch period, ate in twenty minutes, and followed the relaxation routine you've just read about for half an hour before he started back for work.

Result? Two years later, Herman won a trip to Canada for running the best service department in his district.

"Thanks to that noon-hour-break," he told me, "I can keep a smile on my face and some starch in my back all through the day, and still find the energy someplace for a little social life."

Insomnia-combatting relaxation. Once you have learned to relax in the face of normal tensions you can apply the same technique against stresses and worries which are robbing you of sleep. In a sense, loss of sleep is less of a problem than concern about loss of sleep. You toss around in bed frantically repeating to yourself:

"I've got to go to sleep! I won't be worth a hang tomorrow if I don't get to sleep!"

You not only lose sleep, you get absolutely no rest!

If you put part-by-part relaxation to work for you, all this is changed. Actual measurement has shown that energy expenditure declines farther with part-by-part relaxation than with sleep—proof that resting time used in this way is actually more efficient than sleep itself. You don't have to roll and toss and worry about whether you'll be any good in the morning: relax and restore your full capacities, whether you sleep or not! Just follow the basic method described above with one exception: if you find it difficult to relax a whole arm or a whole leg in the face of worry and strain, break down the area to smaller and smaller parts. Relax your hand, your forearm and your upper arm, or even one finger at a time, instead of your whole arm at once.

You can use this technique even if you've always thought of yourself as a born, incurable worry-wart. One of my patients, Peter Sanford, didn't believe that he would ever banish the worry whirl from his sleepless brain.

"I've used sleeping pills for years," he told me. "Whenever I get into a financial hole or have a family argument—anything upsetting—I need medicine to put me to sleep. No matter how I try to control my thoughts, the same old worries and tensions keep popping into my mind."

"Just try this method," I told him. "I'm sure you'll be able to master it."

A few months later, Peter Sanford was back in my office.

"I haven't taken a single sleeping pill for five months," he told me. "That relaxation technique really works! Took me a few weeks to get the hang of it, but I've felt great ever since. Funny thing, when you don't fight to get to sleep, you usually forget your worries and drop off in a hurry, too."

The tension-easing refresher slouch. When you have mastered bedbound relaxation in the face of stresses and worry, you can apply the technique in the upright position to keep tension from building up in the first place. Used in this way, a tension-easing break works wonders for your temperament and your efficiency. Best technique: the refresher slouch.

> Sit in a straight chair with both feet flat on the floor. Let your hands rest relaxed in your lap, with your shoulders sagging forward. Close your eyes and let your head hang loose in front of your chest. Relax as completely as possible, part by part. Continue deliberate relaxation until you cannot feel stiffness or tension anywhere in your body. This usually takes about one minute. Then lift your right hand to shoulder height and let it fall limply into your lap again. Do the same with your left hand. Try to relax part by part even more completely. After another minute, you will find that you are able to take up the cares of the day in a much more relaxed and comfortable way.

How often should you use the tension-breaking refresher slouch? That depends on how much pressure you must withstand. Every housewife should work in a refresher slouch during the hectic presupper hour. Most businessmen need a midmorning and midafternoon break. Some of my patients average almost one break an hour, which still involves no real lost time: they find boosted efficiency and mental calm makes many brief rest breaks worthwhile. Check your own day for tension-ridden hours, and interrupt such periods with two minute breaks. You'll find them very helpful.

Tranquilizing tubs. Next to part-by-part relaxation, the most readily available home remedy for fatiguing irritability and jangled nerves is the tranquilizing tub. This tonic technique works especially well when things are getting you down—when you feel blue and depressed, and life hardly seems worth living. It also helps built-up tension and insomnia. All you need is a bathtub, two towels, some string, and a floating or candy-making thermometer to get considerable relief. Here's how to do it:

> Fill your tub with water at 94 to 98 degrees Fahrenheit. Roll one towel so that it forms a tube with the upper end around the faucet and the lower end trailing in the water. Attach it to the faucet with string or with a strong rubber band. Be sure the overflow drain in the tub works properly. Get into the tub. Turn the water back on, adjusting to a slow flow of lukewarm water. The water flowing into the tub usually has to be kept at about 100 degrees in order to overcome cooling by evaporation and to keep the tub continuously at 94 to 98 degrees. A little experience will soon show what flow and what temperature work the best. When the tub is adjusted, arrange the second towel in a small pillow-like roll and place it behind your neck to support your head as you lie back in relaxed comfort. Stay in the tub for at least a half hour. The soothing effect increases with duration. Many patients find baths up to two or three hours worthwhile, especially when they have been very upset or blue.

Tranquilizing tub treatments can help pull you out of the very depths of gloom. They can also help you shuck off the cares and worries of daily life. Try them: you'll be surprised at how effective they can be.

Wet sheet packs. Wet sheet packs are less easily managed than other home measures against wearying tension or depression because you must induce a member of your family to learn and apply this method before you can enjoy its benefits. The technique is much easier than it sounds, though: after you have gone through the routine once or twice, you will find that you can get into a pack in two minutes or less. The soothing effect helps anyone who has been under extra pressure, and is powerful enough to calm victims of even extreme external or internal strain. If you feel the need for inner peace or uplift, whether from normal living strains or from some severe disturbance, try a wet sheet pack. The only special equipment required is a sheet of plastic, rubber, or oilcloth. You will also use two wool blankets, an ordinary bed sheet, a basin or tub, and your bed. Here's the step by step technique:

Spread a wool blanket on the bed, then a sheet of plastic, rubber, or oilcloth on top. Partly fill a basin with cold water, between 60 and 70 degrees Fahrenheit. Undress and lie on your side at the edge of the bed away from your helper, facing away from him. Have your helper dip the folded sheet in the cold water and wet it thoroughly. Then have him wring it out and spread it quickly along the middle of the bed, the top about one inch from the top of the blanket and the side toward you gathered into lengthwise pleats which will spread easily. Now roll onto the cold, wet sheet. You may shiver for a few moments, but the discomfort will pass quickly. Have your helper spread the sheet completely. Raise your arms above your head. Have your helper wrap one half of the sheet around your body, with its top end high under the armpits. Lower your arms. Have your helper wrap the other half of the sheet around you arms and all, with its upper border diagonal across your chest and its upper corner under the back of your neck. Now have your helper press the sheet down between your legs and fold the end loosely underneath your feet. The sheet should be snug, but not tight.

Next your helper should fold one half of the blanket and its waterproof covering across your body and tuck it in, then the other half. By this time you should be feeling warm and relaxed. Another blanket or two, a pillow or folded towel under your neck, a well-padded hot water bottle near your feet if necessary, and you will enjoy from thirty to sixty minutes of wonderfully complete calm.

One caution: wet sheet packs work well only when they are applied rapidly. It's a good idea to go through a dry run or two with your helper before you wet the sheet: otherwise you will get into your pack so slowly that you will be chilled instead of warmed and relaxed by it.

Soothing massage. Massage is the least available of the great natural tonics because it takes so much practiced assistance. If you are lucky enough to have someone who is willing to learn how to give massage and spend half to three-quarters of an hour giving you each treatment, it is often very soothing. Here's the technique:

Wear loose, easily adjusted clothing such as a nightgown or a pair of shorts. Lie down in a comfortable position, with extra pillows if you need them. Uncover one arm, and have your helper powder it thoroughly with talc. Let your muscles go completely loose: don't try to help in any way. Now your helper should begin slowly and gently stroking the exposed arm, working from the shoulder down. His movements should be perfectly rhythmic, with his hand traveling in a steady oval: down the arm, lift and up again, down the arm, and so on. He should use his other hand to support the arm and to change its position. It is important that the strokes be always in the same direction, and that the massaging hand be gently applied and gently lifted so that there is no sense of jarring at the beginning or end. Your helper's nails should never scratch your skin at the end of a stroke.

The stroking should increase gradually in frequency and vigor as your helper moves along from shoulder to hand, then to the other arm and to the legs. When all the extremities have been massaged, you should turn over.

Similar stroking of the neck and back, this time with both hands at once, makes a good conclusion to massage. The movements should taper to gentle, slow ones as the massage is ended.

Lethargy-fighting tonics. Although tension causes more fatigue than any other factor in American life, some people manage to slough it off without difficulty. In fact, the main complaint many of my patients express is difficulty getting started.

"Nothing bothers me," one of them told me the other day. "In fact, nothing seems to matter much at all. I've felt sometimes that there was something missing—some inner drive or interest or ambition or something—that would really help me make something of my life. But that's just the way I'm built, I guess."

This patient got a tremendous lift out of the next of life's great natural tonics: the *cold friction bath.* Check with your doctor before taking cold friction baths if you have high blood pressure, heart disease, or extreme nervous irritability. Don't take cold baths if you are highly subject to chilblains or to hives brought on by cold exposure. Otherwise, give them a try if you can't get cracking: you'll probably find that cold friction baths make you feel 20 years younger for several hours at a time, and fill you with extra energy and zest. They also often improve your circulation and increase resistance to head colds. The technique is simple and takes little time.

Bundle up well and drink a cup of warm cocoa while you fill your tub. Adjust the temperature of the water to between seventy and eighty degrees Fahrenheit. Undress and get into the bath quickly, immersing your whole body up to the chin. You will gasp for breath for a few moments, but that discomfort will soon pass. If possible, have someone in your family rub the entire surface of your body briskly with both hands all the while you are under the water. Otherwise rub all parts of your own body vigorously yourself with both hands. If the rubbing is sufficiently vigorous, you will feel comfortably warm for from one-half minute to three minutes. Get out of the bath the moment you start to feel chilly. As soon as you get out of the bath, rub yourself briskly with a coarse towel. When as dry as possible, switch to another coarse, dry towel and rub briskly for another two minutes.

Cold friction baths can be made gradually colder and longer as you become accustomed to them. Take them at least twice a week for maximum effect. Lower the temperature about two degrees each time. You will find that you can become accustomed to temperatures down into the fifties if rubbing is sufficiently vigorous.

Home saunas. Anyone who has sweated his way through a home sauna will think I am crazy for saying so, but the main effect comes from *cold* application, not from *hot.* All the ritual of working up a giant sweat simply makes a cold dip or shower comfortable enough to endure. In fact, once the blood is racing through your overheated skin a cold dip or shower feels more like warm honey than ice water, and (except for a bit of initial gasping when each body area is exposed to a new level of cold) you almost never feel chilled with the coldest water flow you can get through your bathroom's pipes.

You have to be able to stand all that stimulation before a sauna is any good to you, and the same limitations cited above for cold friction baths (blood pressure, heart disease, nervous irritability, chilblains, cold-related hives) apply here. There's also very real danger of giddiness or fainting from standing up too quickly while your body is overheated. Warmth opens up all your body's blood vessels, and sudden change of posture can let blood detour to the legs in such quantity that your brain gets no circulation. Best change from lying to sitting to standing only with a considerable pause between stages until your body builds tolerance to heat.

If you observe these limitations, a home sauna can prove a great pick-me-up. Never take a sauna when you have been out in the cold during the last two hours—even brief, mild cold exposure ruins your skin's responsiveness. Sip a little salted broth or Gatorade (or similar product) to avoid heat exhaustion effects, and use a cold towel around the neck if necessary to avoid headache. Sit in the heat until you are sweating all over your body, including your palms and the soles of your feet, which usually takes about twenty minutes—twice as long as it takes to make your face sweat heavily. Move promptly to either a shower or tub for the cold bath part of the program.

If a shower, start with lukewarm water and turn it gradually colder, rubbing with your hands in the area where the water hits and turning to get each part of your body accustomed to every temperature change. You will gasp slightly for breath as the water gets colder, but this will quickly pass. If you get a good blood-vessel reaction, you will feel as if your head is suddenly becoming super-clear. This feeling will usually increase for a minute or two after the bath gets really cold, then reach a stationary plane. At that point, before you begin to feel chilled, get out of the shower and dry yourself briskly, using a second dry towel for a thirty-second rubdown at the end.

If you must use a tub, fill the tub with the coldest water available before your sauna (because you won't have time to fill it afterward). By the time you are ready to use it, the water will have warmed slightly. Follow the procedure described above for cold friction baths, which you will find comfortable with much colder water after working up a good sweat "hot rocks" style.

How to tone up flabby muscles and do-nothing nerves with a sheet bath. If someone in your family will help you, here's a way to tone yourself up with very little mess or bother. You can enjoy the stimulation of a sheet bath with very little equipment or space. Here's how to do it:

> Warm one sheet in your oven beforehand, and put it in the bathroom. Gather another sheet from the ends like a drawn curtain. Soak it in water between 60 and 80 degrees Fahrenheit. Take off your clothes and stand in the bathtub or shower stall, preferably with a rubber bath mat to assure good footing. Have your helper hold up the wet sheet. Raise your arms. Have your helper place an upper corner of the wet sheet in your right armpit. Lower your right arm to hold the sheet in place. Turn to your right, wrapping the sheet around under your left arm and across your back. Drop your other arm and turn until your body is completely enveloped in the sheet. Have your helper tuck in the loose upper corner snugly or pin it to hold the sheet in place. Now your helper should immediately rub your body through the sheet, using long, vigorous strokes down the length of your arms, body, and legs. When your helper feels definite surface warmth through the sheet all over your body, he should unwrap you and put on the dry, warm sheet in exactly the same way. Have him continue rubbing with long, vigorous, lengthwise strokes until you are thoroughly dried.

From the beginning to end, a sheet bath takes four to six minutes. Counting preparation time and clean-up, you'll spend less than ten minutes for a new sensation of tingling liveliness. Try it soon!

Sex as a tonic. In a sense, sex is a fair-weather friend. When things are going well for you and your marriage relations are completely cordial, sex adds boundlessly to your energy, tranquility, and contentment. When you are upset or depressed, or when your marriage is going sour, both your sexual capacities and sexual enjoyment suffer severely. You must often use other natural tonics or even medical measures to get yourself in shape for sex, but once you are ready for relaxed indulgence, you'll reap both soothing and stimulating effects.

Don't let temporary sexual impairments add to your worries or depression. A great many of my patients have encountered this vicious circle: tension or depression upsets their sex life, concern about the disturbed sex life leads to further tension or depression, which upsets sex life further still. These unfortunate people often cannot get their lives back on an even keel until they realize that their sexual capacities are not permanently or seriously impaired. For instance, Bill Farnham complained that he could not maintain an erection.

"I'm only forty-five," he told me despondently. "But I must be in my eighties from the waist down."

Bill's troubles had started a few months before, when his daughter eloped with a young man of whom the Farnhams disapproved. During the period of tension that followed, Bill found himself sexually incapable. He became thoroughly alarmed. Every time he developed designs on his loving wife, he spent the whole evening worrying. "Will I be able to make a go of it tonight?" he would ask himself over and over. No wonder he was too keyed up for sexual success by the time he got ready for bed!

Like most similar sufferers, Bill Farnham regained his capacities almost overnight as soon as he understood the source of his difficulties. Sexual relations call for a complex fusion of physical and emotional factors, which almost any severely upsetting experience can temporarily upset. If you realize that fact, you will not let an occasional failure under duress add further burdens of doubt and fear. You will avoid vicious-circle type sex incapacity.

Tone up for sex when you suffer depression or jitters. The other great natural tonics we have discussed in this chapter do wonders in preparation for sex. There is no better way to start an evening which will culminate in marital communion than with sheet baths or massage. Sex caps the climax of the other tone-up processes. It is the crowning tonic, to be used only after you have soothed or stimulated yourself out of any accumulated tension or the blues.

HOME CORRECTIVES FOR SEVERAL FREQUENT FATIGUING DISORDERS

One of the worst features of fatigue-causing disorders is that people often suffer along with them for years before seeking relief. These problems arise so gradually that victims often think of their low energy store as part of their time of life or as a perfectly normal result of wear and tear. Yet many of these disorders yield quickly to home correctives, and others vanish after inexpensive and painless varieties of prescription care. If you tire more quickly than you think you should, you may find the key to renewed energy and zestful productivity in the next few pages.

How to conquer ordinary low-grade anemia. If the oxygen-carrying strength of your blood is not quite up to its ideal level, you will get a big boost from extra *iron-containing foods.* You should suspect this condition if you tire easily and if your fingernail beds are somewhat paler than those of heartier friends.

Eggs build up your blood. They work especially well if you take them at the same meal with citrus fruits, which help you to digest and make use of egg iron even though they contain little iron themselves. Two eggs with a glass of orange juice should be part of your standard blood-building breakfast.

Meat is another blood builder. A good serving of meat at lunch and at dinner helps fight off borderline anemia. You can use organ meats like liver, heart, and kidneys to keep down the cost if you wish: they are just as effective as expensive steaks and chops.

Iron tablets. Iron pills are also cheap and safe. The best form of iron pills for low grade anemia is ferrous gluconate. It is both cheaper and better than most blood building tonic mixtures. Since iron soaks into your system much more thoroughly when you take it on an empty stomach, you should take three tablets each day, one before each meal. If you are the one person in fifty who gets some heartburn or loss of appetite from ferrous gluconate tablets on this schedule, take them immediately after meals instead. This almost always controls their slight indigestion-spurring effect.

Any form of iron pill may cause your bowel movements to turn black, so don't be alarmed at this change. Some people find iron tablets somewhat constipating: try extra fruit and fluid intake if your pills cause bowel trouble.

Overweight. If you can pinch up a roll of abdominal fat between your thumb and forefinger which is more than one inch thick, you will probably gain substantial extra stores of strength and endurance by losing weight.

"Easier said than done," you say.

That's true. But here are some methods which might help you.

Appetite-spoiling snacks. Properly chosen, snacks can actually help you to lose weight. Overweight patients often digest food in such a way that sugar reaches their bloodstream very slowly. The appetite-control centers in the brain spur the victims to eat more and more, long after a rise in the sugar content of the blood should have occurred to signal "stop." An appetite-spoiling snack starts your blood sugar on the rise ahead of time and helps you to cure excess mealtime appetite. You still have to eat very slowly to allow hunger-killing sugars to reach your brain before you overeat. Sometimes you have to leave the table just a little hungry, with the knowledge that continued soaking up of sugars from inside your stomach and bowel will soon make you completely comfortable. But an appetite-spoiling snack definitely helps.

Like any reduction method, this one has catches. The appetite spoiling snacks have to come *out of* the fuel-or-fat value allowed by an ordinary reduction diet instead of being *added to* it. If you are using a 1000 or 1200 calorie diet or a calorie counting booklet, that means cutting your noon and evening meals by 80 calories each to allow for the calorie content of the recommended snacks. If you are following an exchange system diet, you need to drop two exchanges per meal. Appetite-spoiling snacks work well only if you eat them at exactly the right time, which is not more than one hour or less than forty-five minutes before your noon and evening meals. The variety of allowable foods is not great, but the effect makes snacks worthwhile even if you have to choke them down like medicine.

Here are the snacks my patients usually prefer:

1 hard boiled or soft boiled egg,

or

One-half cup noncreamed cottage cheese, which has a lower fat content than the ordinary creamed variety, but just as much protein.

or

One-quarter cup noncreamed cottage cheese with two tablespoonfuls of reduction-type fruit salad or other fruit.

Most people who are plagued by overweight know the calorie charts and standard diets backwards and have a bureau drawer full of diet sheets. If you are not in that group, you can get a free pamphlet entitled "Overweight and Underweight" which includes complete dietary instructions from the Metropolitan Life Insurance Company, 1 Madison Avenue, New York 10, N.Y.

Reduction-aiding surrender. In helping over two thousand patients toward weight control, I have found this the most important single factor: if they report to someone every week and surrender their food decisions largely to him, they almost always lose satisfactorily. The person to whom they report does not have to be a doctor or even a dietitian. As long as the patient has the feeling that he has put himself into the other person's hands so far as eating is concerned, he loses weight.

In America over 80 per cent of the people gain weight when they are under stress. Overweight people frequently notice this association of stress with overeating: they report that they eat when they feel at loose ends or when they are depressed or upset. Such emotional factors influence your eating behavior *only when you make your own food decisions.* If you have the feeling that somebody else is making those decisions, the mechanism which drives you toward overweight ceases to work. You can put this simple fact to work for you in your own home by getting your husband or wife or closest friend to take over menu planning completely. Arm him with diet sheets and booklets, arrange for him to plan extra snacks for you (subtracting the necessary food values from mealtime allowances) if you complain of hunger or weakness at any one time of the day, then eat exactly as he recommends. Once you have explained your needs, your likes and your dislikes, don't let him put a single food decision into your hands: give him the facts, air your complaints, but let him decide exactly what you should do.

High water intake. When I first started helping patients lose weight, the standard advice was: "Cut down on liquids—try to wring out a few pounds of moisture along with the fat." Now we've gone over to exactly the opposite advice, but to achieve the same end. We've found that if you drink enough *water* it actually *helps* you to wring fat-formed fluid out of your system.

Note that I said *water,* not *liquid.* Where we were making our mistake before was in treating coffee and tea as if they were the same as plain water, which they are not. Coffee and tea actually spur your kidneys artificially to extra urine production, but in a way which proves of no help in moving fluid out of body-burnt fat. Each pound of fat (combined with other body-supplied ingredients) forms two pounds of extra water as it dissolves. Apparently a flood of plain water helps your body unlock this fluid from the fatty tissues, while coffee, tea or cola gives no help (and most other flavored fluids have too much fuel value to include in a low-calorie diet). So drink at least eight glasses of plain water a day while trying to loose weight—you'll be surprised at the result.

Weight-aiding schedule. One final point about overweight: the strain which drives most people to eat ungovernedly is the feeling of being at loose ends and not quite sure what is coming next. Most of my patients do much better on a tight, written schedule. I usually advise scheduling all work, household activity, and plannable recreations. As for free time and social activity, try to write down exactly what you are going to do a day or so in advance. If you can write your diary 24 hours ahead of time and then stick to what it says, you will find yourself under much less psychological pressure to overeat.

Underweight. Underweight people often complain of fatigue, especially late in the morning, afternoon, and evening. The problem here is mainly a lack of fuel reserves. When the calories from your last meal have been exhausted, your muscles and brain have no ready supply of nourishment. You feel dull, depressed, and exhausted.

Either ready fuel supply at the time or the fuel reserves of a few extra pounds will give you tremendous help.

Energizing snacks. If you are underweight, or even if you suffer a late morning and afternoon let-down in spite of normal weight, extra energizing snacks are quite worthwhile. Such snacks produce an actual, measured gain in efficiency of 9.7 per cent. An apple, an orange, a bowl of soup or some milk work just as well as the traditional doughnuts and coffee, and offer extra strength-boosting nutritional values.

The lactose weight gain program. A quickly digested, high sugar snack at the right time will actually increase your appetite for the next meal, thus adding extra mealtime calories as well as its own fuel values to your weight-increasing food supply. When you eat sugar-producing, quickly digested foods, the amount of sugar in your blood increases. Your body uses some of that sugar for quick energy, and lays up more in storage. When the amount of sugar in your blood falls to normal again, your body gradually stops laying up stored supplies. But it can't stop instantly, so your blood sugar level falls well below normal. As long as your blood sugar is below normal, you feel distinctly hungry. This happens for about thirty minutes a little more than an hour after your high-sugar snack or meal.

You need to skip all other between-meals eating, start your meals with the main course, and take rather large amounts of quickly digested carbohydrate to produce substantial weight gain. Four heaping tablespoonfuls of sugar is the average effective dose. However, many patients find that amount of plain sugar unbearably sweet and use milk sugar instead. Milk sugar, sold in any drugstore under the chemical name "lactose," gives the same appetite-boosting effect as ordinary sugar, but it is only one-eighth as sweet. Lactose which is pure enough for food use (you don't need expensive chemically pure or technical grade) is fairly cheap. You'll find it pleasant to take, too: just stir four heaping tablespoonfuls into tart fruit juice, lemonade, or plain water. Timed exactly one and a half hours before lunch and supper, this dose puts ten pounds onto the average patient in less than a month.

Fatigue from testicular congestion. You can cure fatigue from testicular congestion with very simple home measures. If you have an extra tangle of veins just above the left testicle as big as a walnut or larger, you may be suffering fatigue from testicular congestion. If so, extra scrotal support will definitely increase your strength and energy.

Suspensory. A comfortable elastic scrotal support or suspensory relieves testicular congestion at a cost of a dollar or so. Wear a suspensory for a couple of weeks. If it makes you more energetic and less easily fatigued, buy several suspensories and wear one all the time. Otherwise, put your suspensory in the bureau drawer and try again in a year or so: this form of fatigue is so gradual in onset that often the only way you know it is there is by the relief you get from suspensory support.

Fatigue from sexual over-indulgence. An overdose of any tranquilizer leads to torpor, albeit blissful torpor. Sex is no exception. Despite old wives' tales which blame sex-weariness on diet, the plain fact seems to be that it is due to an imbalance in your sympathetic nervous system with over-action of the anti-excitement, anti-stimulation element.

Alternate hot-cold showers. You can often bring the elements of your sympathetic nervous system back into balance after sexual over-indulgence with alternate hot-cold showers. Start with fairly hot water, spraying every part of your body surface. Rub vigorously with both hands in the area being sprayed. Adjust the water to as much heat as you can stand, then abruptly switch to a cold spray. Continue vigorous rubbing until gasping subsides, turning to expose all body parts. The cold spray will then feel comfortable for twenty to thirty seconds. Before you start to feel chilled, switch back to hot water for two minutes or so. Continue alternating hot and cold for about ten minutes, then rub yourself briskly all over with a succession of dry, coarse towels.

Types of fatigue for which your doctor's help is worthwhile. Severe fatigue certainly deserves medical care just as much as disabling pain or other miseries. However, even mild fatigue may point to conditions for which prompt medical care will prove worthwhile. If you know what accompanying signs to watch out for, you will detect the underlying cause of your fatigue sooner and win relief much more quickly than if you wait until severe difficulty drives you to your doctor's office.

Blood loss anemia. If you can stop the loss of a few drops of blood each day, you relieve your blood-forming organs of a great strain. The blood loss may not be alarming—I've had patients who didn't think it was even worth mentioning. But you often gain stronger blood and extra energy by stopping any form of persistent bleeding.

Here are several types of continual bleeding which you may be able to spot, and which your doctor can usually stop with inexpensive and painless measures:

1. Heavy or long-lasting menstrual flow. Periods should last no more than seven days, and should soil about one dozen pads per month. Heavier flow or passage of frequent or large clots deserves medical correction.

2. Bleeding with stools, even if it obviously comes from hemorrhoids.

3. One or more black, bulky stools, especially if they occur after a sudden weak spell. Bleeding into the stomach or intestine often shows up this way because the blood turns black during digestion.

4. Vomiting of bloody or coffee-grounds-like material. Stomach acids change blood into brownish flakes.

5. Frequent or severe nosebleeds.

6. Reddish or blood-tinged urine.

Pernicious anemia. Pernicious anemia resists iron treatment or diet completely, but gets well very promptly with liver or vitamin B_{12} shots. Liver shots might be of tremendous help to you if weakness and tiredness come along with dizzy spells, easy loss of wind, and numbness or tingling of the legs. A tendency to stumble in the dark or to bark your shins frequently also points toward this ailment.

How to conquer fatigue due to a sluggish thyroid. Thyroid hormone makes sluggish body processes speed up. It bestirs energy, keeps your skin and hair healthy, and helps you toward comfortable warmth. Hundreds of thousands of women and tens of thousands of men have found boundless energy in a few cents' worth of thyroid pills a month. These happy people completely, comfortably, and inexpensively replace the thyroid gland products which their own body fails to supply. If you have signs of thyroid deficiency, thyroid pills may offer a safe, inexpensive, and comfortable road to a newly energized life.

When should you suspect thyroid deficiency? If you have three or more of these signs:

1. Dry skin.

2. Coarse or thinning hair.

3. Easy fatigue.

4. Unusual menstruation, either scanty, irregular, heavy, or frequent.

5. Continuous puffiness of eyelids and cheeks (usually so gradual in onset that victims only notice it when they compare their present appearance with old snapshots).

6. Irritability.

7. Sleepiness or sluggishness.

8. Easy chilling—victims often want the room much warmer than other people, and need extra sweaters and extra covers.

Lila Grant found boundless energy and new calm and contentment through thyroid pills. Tension crackled between Lila Grant and her husband, Bill, when they first came to my office.

"For the last three or four years," Bill said, "Lila's been getting worse and worse. She's so irritable it's driving all of us nuts. There must be *something* wrong—she wasn't that way before."

Lila's face was pinched under coarse, dull hair. Her dry-skinned, rough hands were in tight fists.

"I don't know," she said. "Maybe there is something wrong. I fly off the handle over nothing, and I know I shouldn't. But what can I do?"

Tests showed that Lila needed thyroid pills. A few months later, Bill came to my office with her again.

"Lila's got her disposition back again, doctor," he said. "It's simply wonderful what those pills do for her."

That's what most patients say, and their families, too. Whether thyroid lack causes sluggishness or irritability or both, it always causes misery. A few visits to a doctor do a world of good.

How to conquer fatigue from overactive thyroid. An overactive thyroid can be tamed with medicines or surgically removed. Left alone, it makes body processes race at an inefficient rate. If you have an overactive thyroid, your heart races and pounds. You sweat a great deal and feel uncomfortably warm. You lose weight in spite of good appetite. You become nervous and irritable.

An overactive thyroid is usually swollen. You can see definite fullness or a lump a couple of inches down from your Adam's apple. The fullness moves up and down with the Adam's apple when you swallow.

Your doctor can give worthwhile help if you have an overactive thyroid. See him soon if you suspect that this is troubling you.

How to avoid diabetes. Some people can avoid diabetes entirely by discovering and correcting their tendency toward the disease. If you are more than twenty pounds overweight, or if your family background includes many victims of diabetes or of overweight, special tests for diabetic tendencies may be worthwhile. Here's a case which shows what you might accomplish:

When Doris Maxwell was 43, her younger sister developed diabetes. Doris decided she should have a thorough checkup herself, since her mother and brother also suffered the same disease.

Doris did not have diabetes, but her tests showed an abnormal blood-sugar curve. This meant that she was fated for that disease soon, unless she took steps to avoid it. Doris immediately began to eat more meat and eggs and less sugars and starches. Her special diet is not at all hard to follow—no measured quantities or rigid menus. She uses low-calorie substitutes for sugar wherever possible and omits excess sweets and starches. For very little money or inconvenience she has kept herself entirely free of diabetes. In fact, she now has a completely normal blood-sugar curve, and is one stage further away from disease than she was five years ago.

How to hold diabetes in check. Even if you do not avoid diabetes altogether, you can probably avoid its ravages. Your doctor can help you to live out virtually your full lifespan in comfort and efficiency. He can keep you from suffering the complaints which victims of uncontrolled diabetes endure. He can slow down the rapid aging to which diabetics are prone.

Every day that diabetes remains unchecked, its victim ages several days to a week. What a terrible waste, when a few cents' worth of medicine a day could stop unduly rapid deterioration! If you fall victim to diabetes, you can keep vigor and strength for many extra years by finding and caring for your disorder promptly.

How can you find it promptly? Most patients complain mainly of fatigue and frequent infections like colds, boils and festering sores. Many lose weight in spite of a good appetite, or eat vast amounts without weight gain. Constant thirst is a tip-off, along with increased urination. But many victims of diabetes never realize that anything serious is wrong until a urine test shows extra sugar. If you're in that group, you could profit tremendously from one new development: home urine-testing kits are now distributed free at drug stores almost everywhere during Diabetes Detection Week (the third week in November). Or you can buy test materials and directions for a few cents per test and check a sample voided about two hours after your main meal. A positive test does not always mean diabetes, but it does mean that you should get your doctor to do further examinations. If you find diabetes early, you'll often restore energy you've forgotten you ever had, and at the same time add many years to your life.

CHAPTER THIRTEEN

How to Improve Your Circulation with Home Measures

When my patients start to talk yearningly of retirement to Florida or California, I can usually bet that they suffer substantial circulatory miseries. While Minnesotans grouse about six months of winter, few would trade their four seasons for a one-season year so long as their arteries carry enough warming blood out to their fingertips and their veins let them stomp through the snow without agonizing calf cramps. Activity-limiting effects of poor circulation make winter seem more fierce, whether from varicose veins, phlebitis, dizzy spells, cold hands and feet, or blood-lack leg cramps. Home remedies and correctives can hold all of these conditions at bay, though. Several tried and true techniques will help you to keep both your veins and your arteries working well and to recognize and combat circulatory conditions which account for more hospital operations and more lost limbs than any other disease in the world. Let's start with the commonest, most easily identified conditions, and then move on to the other frequent complaints stemming from diseases of veins or arteries.

HOME MEASURES AGAINST VARICOSE VEINS

Home measures alone may entirely cure small varicose veins. You can control the misery which larger veins cause, slow their growth, and prevent many of their complications with home measures.

How to tell if you have varicose veins. You can check yourself for varicose veins without a doctor's help. Bare your legs and stand perfectly still for about three minutes beforehand. Use a single lamp for a light source. Examine the portion of the leg where the light strikes tangentially, just where the leg's curve makes it fall into shadow. Turn slightly or move the light to bring other areas into vein-revealing focus. Any vein in the lower leg larger than a lead pencil indicates that vein valves have given way. More advanced varicosities show up as winding, enlarged surface veins. Tiny sunbursts of surface veins need not be considered: your doctor can eliminate them with injection treatments if you wish, but they do not cause circulatory problems.

Home measures can stop the formation or growth of varicose veins. You can keep small, beginning varicose veins from growing larger and keep new varicosities from forming by controlling or interrupting leg vein engorgement. Ordinarily, the calf muscles squeeze on the deep leg veins with each leg motion and send a spurt of blood up along the main leg veins. When the muscles relax, the deep veins fill with blood from the surface veins. Valves prevent the blood from backing up into surface veins during muscle contraction, and still allow it to flow freely at other times. These valves look like shirt pockets sewed lengthwise to the inside of the veins. When the blood flows from the surface to the deep veins, it goes past each pocket from the closed end. When the blood tries to flow from the deep to the surface veins, it runs into the open end of the pocket-like valve which fills and balloons out into the vein passage. Each valve pocket is barely big enough to stop up the vein at its ordinary size. If you stand or sit still for a long time, the vein may become engorged and stretch until it is too large for its valves to close off. Blood backing up from the deep veins stretches the surface and connecting veins further. This leads both to the unsightly, wormlike surface varicosities, and to breakdown of more and more vein valves.

You can usually stop varicosity formation completely by taking these three steps:

1. Eliminate vein-engorging constrictions and pressures. Free flow of blood from the leg veins to the heart makes valve-impairing engorgement much less likely. Main measures which help to guarantee free flow: use a garter belt or girdle instead of round or elastic garters. Wear loose-fitting clothing which does not bind at the knee or thigh for sustained or strenuous work and play.

2. Pump blood out of your leg veins frequently with muscular action during prolonged sitting or standing. From either sitting or standing posture, rock up on your heels, lifting the toes of both feet as high as possible. Return to normal position. Rock up on your toes. Return to normal position. Repeat three times every 20 to 30 minutes.

3. Flush veins thoroughly with the aid of gravity drainage every two hours during prolonged sitting or standing. This exercise is a great refresher, whether you have normal leg veins or varicosities. Take off your shoes. Lie on your back, and bring your legs up until your knees are directly above your head. Stretch your legs and feet straight up, bracing your hips with your hands. (Alternate method: lie with hips on the arm of an overstuffed davenport and with legs stretched straight up.) With feet and ankles entirely relaxed, jiggle the legs with short, rapid to-and-fro motions. The flopping about of the foot milks fatigue-causing wastes out of the muscles and flushes the leg veins thoroughly in about 30 seconds.

How to control varicose vein miseries. If you have lead-pencil-size varicosities, they probably cause more fatigue and discomfort than you realize. Varicose veins make your feet and legs tire very quickly, lead to frequent foot and leg cramps, and sometimes impair circulation to the skin of the lower leg so badly that it becomes congested or develops open sores. Varicose veins decrease the effective circulation in the other, deep-lying veins of the leg without in any way replacing it. When the leg musculature squeezes on the deep leg veins, they squirt blood past the ineffective surface vein valves into the stretched, stagnant varicosities instead of toward the heart. When the leg musculature relaxes, blood from the varicose backwash pours back into the deep veins. The muscles and other tissues get only a fraction of the circulation they deserve because the deep vein pumping action is wasted on back-and-forth movement of stagnant blood.

Gravity-aided vein flushing. With mild varicose veins—enlargement, but no tortuosity—gravity-drainage vein flushing usually keeps varicose veins from impairing the circulation in your legs. The communicating veins in such cases are usually not so badly stretched that their valves do not work at all: the valves only fail when the veins become engorged. Frequent vein flushing keeps engorgement from occurring. Follow the gravity-aided vein flushing program described above every two hours throughout the day, and every hour during periods when you are usually standing or sitting still.

Elastic bandages. Elastic bandages keep most varicosities from impairing your circulation. Smooth, steady pressure from the outside keeps surface veins from absorbing the blood that should push on toward the heart. Get a four-inch elastic bandage (two lengths if any veins above the knee are enlarged). The rubberized bandages give snugger support than plain cotton, although some patients must use plain cotton because rubber irritates their skin. Keep the remaining bandage rolled as you apply each turn, and stretch the bandage about halfway to its maximum length as you wind it on. Apply two anchor turns around the ankle. Carry the bandage down from the front of the ankle for a turn around the foot. Now spiral up the leg, overlapping approximately half the width of the bandage on each turn. If more than one length of bandage is needed to extend above the highest engorged vein, fasten the end of the first bandage with the hooks provided or with safety pins, then start another bandage with one or two turns overlapping the first bandage and spiral on up the leg. When you reach the knee, bandage with the joint partly bent and take two or three Figure-8 turns—one loop below the knee, one above, joining at the back of the joint. Continue your spiral and fasten the bandage top as before.

Long underwear. Many patients (even women) find that the easiest way to keep a bandage in place is to wear long cotton knit underwear underneath it. If you do this, you can draw the bandage somewhat tighter. Be sure that the knit fits snugly enough to be relatively free of wrinkles and folds.

Periodic leg exercises. An elastic bandage allows normal muscle movement to push blood along toward the heart. However, it does not increase the efficiency of circulation while you are sitting still or standing. You should get in the habit of pumping the blood out of your leg veins every few minutes when you are standing or sitting still by rocking up on your toes and heels alternately.

Take a few days' home treatment for varicose veins even if you think they aren't hurting you. Leg aching and fatigue from poor venous circulation come on so gradually that victims often do not realize how much trouble their enlarged leg veins are causing. As one of my patients told me:

"Until I got my veins fixed, I thought aching feet and weariness were just part of getting old. When your feet and legs wear out, you feel worn out all over. But it just doesn't happen like that any more. I can keep going all day, and then some!"

Try a full-scale program for vein misery control if you have varicose veins, whether you think they are causing you trouble or not. You might be surprised at how much energy and comfort you can restore. I've seen dozens of patients lose complaints they thought were due to old age through simple vein care.

When your doctor can give worthwhile help for varicose veins. Even in cases formerly ruled as incurable, modern surgical techniques almost always give permanent relief for varicose vein suffering. If any of your lower leg veins is bigger than a lead pencil, you should discuss the problem with your doctor during your next visit.

The presence or imminent danger of open sores is a more pressing reason for getting medical care for varicosities. Open sores usually form on the outer side of the leg just above the ankle. Redness, itching, and scaling or brownish discoloration in this area usually precede ulcer formation by several weeks or months. Any of these signs in combination with moderately severe or severe varicose veins should send you to your doctor in a hurry. With prompt attention, you may save yourself the misery of a months-long smoldering infection.

Although most experts today prefer operation to injection treatment, a permanent cure for varicose veins involves much less disability and discomfort than most people think. One or two days in the hospital and a few more days at home usually solves your vein problem for good. The procedure causes much less pain than any abdominal operation. The biggest barrier is cost, which is usually about the same (for both legs) as for an appendectomy.

HOW TO WARD OFF PHLEBITIS

You can frequently keep raw or clot-plugged veins from troubling you by taking simple measures at home. If phlebitis does strike, you can often avoid serious risks by deciding promptly what is wrong and taking the proper steps.

How to prevent fireman's phlebitis. Most firemen freely admit to poor physical condition. For weeks on end, they sit around the station playing pinochle and leaning on a polishing rag. Then comes a four alarm fire and they run up and down ladders like a bunch of boy scouts in a relay race. No wonder two or three men show up with phlebitis after each major fire! Unaccustomed, prolonged exertion plays havoc with delicate veins. However, our Minnesota hunters and outdoorsmen have found three rules which help them to keep clear of this problem:

1. Train up to heavy exertion. Take a walk each evening in the weeks before hunting season, practice a few minutes every day for a week or two before you try your first 18 holes of golf.

2. Bracket periods of exertion between a good warm-up and a slow tapering of activity. One of my patients always walks several blocks to the tennis courts and back, for instance. He's still good for three sets at age eighty-two.

3. Use elastic bandages for extra vein support if these steps are impossible.

How to dodge the phlebitis of immobility. The phlebitis of immobility is next in susceptibility to home measures. Whenever you go to bed for several days without getting up or moving around, your circulation becomes quite sluggish. Especially in your older years, the risk that slow-flowing blood will clot in the veins of the legs or pelvis is quite real. You can avoid this hazard by following two rules:

1. Never stay in bed continuously without consulting your physician. Complete bed rest is a very dangerous treatment unless precautions are taken against phlebitis. Even if you're sure you'll soon get well, an illness which keeps you from getting up to eat and to toilet yourself deserves medical care.

2. When you stay in bed with a cold or other minor illness, make it a point to change your position in bed every fifteen minutes while you are awake. Roll on one side, then the other. Prop yourself up on several pillows, then let yourself back down. Exactly the same principle holds when you are under a doctor's care. If your physician doesn't give you specific orders about moving around in bed, be sure to ask him what you should do. Moving in bed is especially important after surgical operation and obstetric delivery, so take special care to keep mobile at such times.

How to interrupt migratory phlebitis. The form of phlebitis next most likely to yield to home measures is clotting of the veins underneath the skin. People who are subject to such attacks get them repeatedly, in different parts of the body. Each vein heals into a firm, non-tender strand in ten days to three weeks.

You can make further attacks of surface vein clotting much less likely to occur if you discontinue the use of tobacco. Since this condition is sometimes a vanguard of other more serious circulatory problems, this step is well worthwhile. If will power alone won't get you free of the smoking habit, try Chapter 15's suggested techniques.

How to ward off infectious phlebitis. The last form of phlebitis which you can avoid through home measures is due to involvement of the vein walls in the spread of infection from a surface sore. The techniques for controlling skin infections which we discussed on page 145 will keep this kind of spread from occurring.

How to spot phlebitis before serious complications occur. Most serious vein clots occur in the deep veins of the lower leg. Every movement of the calf muscles presses on these veins, so you suffer some discomfort on walking and on tipping the foot upward. Pain is never severe, however, and is sometimes barely noticeable. The blocked vein passages lead to slight swelling of the ankle and foot. Some patients have a degree or so of fever.

Phlebitis in surface veins or varicosities makes the vessels firm and tender, usually with some reddening of the skin above them. Your doctor can use medicines to keep the clot from spreading into the deep veins if you call him promptly.

HOW TO CONTROL DIZZY SPELLS

You can sort out several types of dizziness through simple home tests and observations. You can get substantial, lasting relief from many of these conditions with little or no expense or discomfort through home care. You can decide promptly which spells call for a doctor's care. Here's a step by step program for handling dizzy spells which covers all of these points:

What to do when dizziness strikes. Lie down perfectly flat with your eyes closed and your head stationary. While the dizziness continues, check these points to help guide your management of future attacks:

Do you seem to whirl, or does the room whirl around you?
Do you get worse when you move your head?
Is your breathing deeper or more constrained than usual?
If you can feel your pulse, is it rapid or slow?

After the attack subsides, consider the answers to these four questions and the circumstances in which the dizziness occurred. Try to determine which of these forms of dizziness plagues you, and take appropriate action:

Balance organ dizziness. If the room seems to be whirling around you, your dizziness is probably due to sensitivity of the balance organ inside of your ear or irritation of the nerves connected with that organ. Further confirmatory test: moving your head rapidly from side to side will make you temporarily worse, and sometimes will also make you sick to your stomach. Effective home measures:

1. Nose drops, ¼ per cent neosynephrine or ½ per cent ephedrine in isotonic saline (available in many states without prescription, and perfectly safe for everyone except victims of severe heart disease or high blood pressure). Lie with your head over the side of the bed, lower than the level of your chest, turn your head to one side, and put two drops in the lower of the two nostrils. After 30 seconds, turn your head the other way and put two drops in the other nostril. Repeat every four hours for two days.

2. A low salt diet, which is usually needed for at least six weeks. No salty foods like ham or patato chips, no salt added either in preparation or at table to other foods.

3. Motion sickness pills, either Dramamine or Bonamine, which you can get at any drug store without prescription.

These measures have only about a fifty-fifty chance of bringing the attacks of dizziness under control. If they fail to bring about marked improvement inside two days, you should see your doctor.

Overbreathing-type dizziness. One type of dizziness almost always responds to home measures: overbreathing alkalosis. The attack starts with giddiness and light-headedness, usually accompanied by tingling of the hands, feet, and sometimes the face. In severe cases, muscle spasms make the hands draw up and the toes curl. The initial light-headedness gradually goes on to frank whirling sensations. This series of complaints is actually due to rapid, deep breathing. Such breathing blows off an essential portion of your blood's main acid substance, leaving the body alkalies in full control.

Rebreathing. If you hold the opening of a large plastic bag snugly against your face and breathe in and out of it, overbreathing type dizziness will usually abate. Rebreathe the same air for two or three minutes, even though it seems to be getting stuffy. Empty the bag of old air and start rebreathing again immediately if symptoms are not entirely under control.

Breath holding. You can usually nip attacks in the bud by holding every other breath at the first sign of giddiness or tingling. Continue for six to ten breaths, or until symptoms abate.

How to manage fainting type dizziness. Some dizzy spells are simply a mild form of fainting. Sudden giddiness during an emotional crisis, at the sight of blood, or in the presence of pain is due to emotional reaction in the blood vessels, detouring blood that would otherwise supply the brain through vessels leading to the muscles and abdominal organs. The blood-starved brain seems awhirl. If you lie flat or sit with your knees spread wide apart and put your head far down between them, the attack usually passes off.

Posture change dizziness. When you stand up, the arteries in your legs have to get very much smaller and the arteries in your neck quite a bit bigger. Otherwise, the blood goes to your feet, leaving your brain poorly supplied. Your arteries may not make these adjustments instantly when you sit or stand quickly. You become lightheaded from lack of circulation to the brain. No serious disorder is responsible. The complaints usually disappear if you sit down and put your head between your knees. People who are subject to this complaint should get in the habit of sitting on the side of the bed for a few moments in the morning and getting up deliberately whenever they have been sitting in the same position for a long time.

Carotid sinus dizziness. If dizzy spells on position change develop in later life, especially if the pulse is markedly slowed during each attack, the chances are that sensitivity of the artery-controlling nerve centers in the neck is at fault. These centers are located on the main neck arteries approximately at the level of the top of your voice box. If they become oversensitive, any position change or any slight pressure over the carotid sinus area can throw you into a severe faint.

One of my patients had this type of difficulty. He had attacks almost every Sunday for months. Problem: the high, starched collar which he only wore for church services rubbed the carotid sinus area. Since he's switched to soft-collared sports shirts, he hasn't had a single attack.

If you think carotid sinus sensitivity might be your trouble, test yourself for it in your own home. Lie down, turn your head slightly to the right, and press the ball of your right thumb against the pulsating artery just to the left of your windpipe, opposite the top of the voice box. Roll the thumb around the surrounding area slightly. If dizziness occurs, release the pressure immediately. If the left sinus proves insensitive, wait at least three minutes before testing the right one. Never under any circumstances press on both sinuses at once.

You will probably find that you can control your complaints by wearing soft open collars and avoiding sudden position change even if your carotid sinuses are quite sensitive. If these measures fail, your doctor can arrange to snip the oversensitive nerves. This operation is quite minor and leaves no serious after-effects, but it almost always gives permanent and lifelong cure.

Low blood-sugar dizziness. Giddy spells, dizziness, or actual faints can stem from a low blood-sugar level. Your brain has no reserve supply of fuel, and blanks out when the blood fails to supply its needs. Usually this problem arises when you have skipped breakfast or gone without food for 12 hours or more. Excitement or tension may also play a part. In some susceptible individuals, attacks occur in the rebound phase an hour or two after any heavy carbohydrate meal (such as waffles with syrup). A soft mint, sugar cube, or glass of sweetened orange juice gives almost instant relief. Victims of frequent attacks can usually avoid trouble by eating snacks between meals and taking meat, eggs, or cottage cheese with each meal for extra slow-burning protein.

Dizziness from medicines. A number of medicines can cause dizziness in people who are unusually subject to their action. Aspirin and the aspirin family, nose drops, nerve quieters, antihistamines, codeine-containing cough syrups and many other common remedies may be at fault. If dizzy spells develop while you are taking any home remedy, discontinue it for two days to see whether the dizzy spells disappear. If dizzy spells develop while you are taking medically prescribed remedies, telephone your doctor.

When your doctor can give worthwhile help for dizzy spells. You need your doctor's help to discover and treat any possibly serious underlying disorder if your dizzy spells are accompanied by other complaints or alterations in body function. Victims of anemia usually complain of fatigue as well as dizziness. High blood pressure causes headaches, loss of wind, and other difficulties along with dizziness. Heart disease almost always causes pain, weakness, or breathlessness before it causes dizziness. Severe diarrhea or vomiting leads to dizzy spells through upset in body salt and fluid balance. Internal bleeding from an ulcer or other condition may cause dizzy spells along with weakness, black, tar-colored stools, and cold sweats. Your doctor can give you substantial help for each of these conditions.

HOME MEASURES FOR COLD HANDS AND FEET AND FOR BLOOD-LACK LEG CRAMPS

You can take several effective steps to combat sluggish blood flow through your arms and legs. The commonest complaint from poor circulation is a sort of cold numbness of the hands and feet. With more severe involvement, patients in the late thirties, forties, and fifties complain mainly of circulation-stopping spasms brought on by cold exposure. Their fingertips turn blue and become very painful whenever their hands become slightly chilled. Older patients are less subject to spasm and more subject to muscle cramps. At first, pain in the calves of the legs occurs only after very prolonged walking or running. As time goes on, the amount of exertion required to bring on an attack steadily decreases, until some victims can only walk half a block or so without pausing to rest. Proper home treatment often boosts circulation enough to vanquish these complaints.

Hot towels to the adjacent trunk area. You can increase the circulation to any important body part with heat, but YOU MUST NEVER APPLY HEAT DIRECTLY TO PARTS IN WHICH CIRCULATION IS IMPAIRED. The trick is to warm the trunk area which shares nerves and blood vessels with the affected part instead of warming the part itself. This makes the blood vessels to the affected area open up without increasing the affected tissue's need for oxygen and fuel, as direct hot applications would do. Before age sixty, most circulatory problems have an element of spasm which can be relieved promptly by hot applications to the upper part of the extremity and to the adjoining trunk. Especially if the attack has been aggravated or brought on by exposure to cold, by emotional upset or by excessive smoking, hot towels to the shoulders and upper arms or to the thighs and hips are worthwhile. Dip the towels in water at 112 degrees, wring partly dry, put them on, and cover with a sheet of plastic or with a dry towel to cut cooling from evaporation.

Warm flannel. After age sixty, gentle, more sustained warmth will gradually bring comfort and improved circulation. Wrap the affected part in warmed flannel or put on long cotton or wool underwear. Use a cushioned heating pad set for low heat across the shoulders or hips. Keep the rest of the body comfortably warm, since heat-induced sweating may make you somewhat subject to chill.

Smoking and circulation. Nicotine increases arterial spasm as long as arteries retain their elasticity. Circulatory difficulties which strike before age sixty, and especially those involving painful blue fingers or abruptly freezing toes, are often greatly improved if you quit smoking. You'll find a helpful home routine to aid you in this difficult task in Chapter Fifteen of this book.

How to boost your circulation with home exercises. You can substantially improve the circulation in your legs with Buerger-Allen vascular exercises if you are plagued by coldness, numbness, or cramps. These exercises are very easy to perform right in your own home. The object is to stretch and stimulate the tiny blood vessels in which the greatest resistance to blood flow occurs by alternately overfilling and draining them. Plan to do Buerger-Allen exercises three times a day for at least three months before you decide how much good they are doing: effects are sometimes slow, but usually prove worthwhile if you persevere. Here are step by step directions:

1. Turn a straight chair over on the lower half of your bed, so that the legs of the chair stick out over the foot of the bed and the chair's back forms an angled platform for your legs when you lie down. Pad the back of the chair with a folded sheet. Lie down on your back with your legs lying along the inclined chair back. Remain in this position for two minutes.

2. Sit up with your feet dangling over the side of the bed. Slowly and deliberately carry out each possible foot and toe motion: turn your toes down, raise them up, turn your feet inward, turn them outward, spread your toes, and close them again. Continue these motions for three minutes.

3. Lie flat in the bed with your feet and legs wrapped in warm blankets. Relax in this position for five minutes.

How Dave Porter improved his waning circulation. Dave Porter's case shows what Buerger-Allen exercises can do.

"I've always thought it was better to wear out than to rust out," Dave told me. "But I'll be blamed if I can keep going any longer! When I try to mow the lawn I can put in just about three turns around the yard, then that's it. Leg cramps! Get so I just can't stand up any more."

Dave was sixty-two, but from the knees up he looked and acted like a man in his late forties. Only the arteries in his legs seemed to be markedly hardened, but one look at the dull, mottled skin of his ankles and feet proved that he was only a few months away from a case of gangrene. I recommended exercises, but with great fear that they would prove futile.

A year later, Dave Porter marched with his lodge brothers on a two and a half mile parade without a spasm or cramp. Buerger-Allen exercises—exactly the same as the ones you can do in your own home without a penny in medical expense—had helped him to unclog his blood vessels. He has remained active for several years now without further difficulty.

Further aids to circulation. If home measures fail to restore circulation, your doctor can suggest many other highly effective techniques. You should never settle for a life hedged about with circulatory limitations simply because people have always talked about these things as immutable burdens. Your doctor can arrange diet and medicines. He can help you to rent inexpensive circulation-stimulating equipment which you can use right in your own home. One hopeful fact: I have never seen and never expect to see a person robbed of a limb by gangrene without months and months of warning symptoms. Pale, lifeless color, sometimes with dry flaking of the skin, coldness to the touch and loss of feeling are good reasons to get your doctor's help. Blood-lack calf cramps, cold feet, and mottling are even earlier warning signs. If you remain alert for lack of circulation, you can bring a legion of home measures and medical aid into the battle to prevent gangrene.

CHAPTER FOURTEEN

How to Make Your Heart and Arteries Last Longer

Too many people are afraid of long life. Age means misery and disability to them: steady decline to a pitiful remnant of their former selves. How wrong these pessimists have proved! Science today can promise that if you combat and hold off the heart and artery diseases which are our most deadly plagues, you will not suffer the miseries and disabilities which people have always blamed on old age. You will add *youthful, vigorous* years to your life.

This is no idle dream. Although further discoveries will certainly shed more light, you can already get effective aid from thoroughly known facts in meeting every one of these life and death problems:

How to win speedier, more complete recovery if a heart attack strikes.
How to get extra help from your doctor for heart and artery troubles.
How to cure frightening but innocent chest pains.
How to fend off hardening of the arteries.
How to avoid coronary heart attacks.
How to keep your blood pressure down.

You can apply the main measures in each of these crucial spheres right in your own home. Here are exact directions.

HOW TO WIN SPEEDIER, MORE COMPLETE RECOVERY IF A HEART ATTACK SHOULD STRIKE YOU

Better than four out of five people who suffer a heart attack get back to full time work and a potentially happy life afterwards. Most of the rest recover well enough to be happy and useful again. If a heart attack strikes you or someone you love, you can do a lot to hold down damage. The outcome of an attack often depends on what is done in the first few minutes, when the doctor hasn't yet arrived. Here's how to handle each of the two main kinds of heart attack when it first strikes:

Painful attacks can best be fought flat, right where they occur. A coronary heart attack strikes with crushing pain in the middle of the chest. The pain may run down the arms or up into the neck. Dizziness and a cold sweat often follow.

Rest and calm. When such an attack strikes, the victim needs rest above all! Absolute rest of body, with all the emotional and mental calm he can muster. Heart experts claim that coronary victims shouldn't be moved from the place of their attack for at least one hour, and often not for two hours or more. A doctor should be at the victim's side, of course. The victim needs relief of pain, which only a doctor can bring. But the doctor can come to the victim's side without sacrificing the crucial help of total rest, while a wild ambulance ride might do terrible harm.

Here's how Pete Armstrong helped himself through a heart attack: Pete Armstrong woke in the middle of the night, fighting for air against the frightful pressure in his chest. He clutched at the lamp on the bedside table, which crashed down to the floor. His wife woke with a start.

"What's wrong?" she said.

Pete only gasped. She reached out to him. Her hand struck the dank coldness of his face.

"My God!" she said, and leaped for the light switch.

"It must be my heart," Pete gasped. "There's a pain in my chest and down my left arm."

"I'll call an ambulance, right away," his wife said.

"No," Pete said, raising his hand. "First get me blankets. I'm supposed to lie quiet, and I'm so cold I'm shivering."

His wife got the extra covers.

"Now call the doctor," Pete said. "But don't just say to come out and hang up. Ask him what we should do now." He closed his eyes and lay quiet. Relaxing in the face of fear and pain was the hardest job he'd ever tackled. He did his best.

"The doctor's coming," his wife said, back at his side. "He says you're doing fine. Just stay relaxed."

That's just what Pete did, as best he could. He spent as little effort as possible, physically, mentally, and emotionally. That fact, more than what his doctor did for him, helped him to recover quickly and completely.

Smothering type heart attacks. Suppose the heart victim doesn't have chest pain. Instead he wakes up at night choking for breath. Or he finds that he needs to stop after every slight exertion to catch his breath, and finally can't breathe naturally even when he's holding still.

Such smothering spells usually come from heart trouble. However, you can still have long years of fully useful, happy, and contented life when they strike.

A lazy, chair-borne ride. A quick, effortless trip to oxygen and medical aid is the key to prompt cure for smothering-type heart attacks. That's what a heart victim needs, and it's usually easy for him to get without paying ambulance fees. The sitting posture is better than the lying one, anyway, and it takes less time to load up and leave than to call for help.

How Muriel Johnson pulled herself through a smothering style heart attack. Muriel Johnson shook her head. She just couldn't get her breath. Middle of the night or not, she had to have help. She called her brother.

"What's wrong?" her brother asked when he burst in.

"It's my heart, I believe," Muriel said. "Don't get upset, though: The doctor warned me that this might happen, and told me what to do."

"He'll come right out?"

"No, he'll meet us at the hospital. Call him for me now. Then get some help and carry me down the stairs. I'm supposed to stay right in this straight chair. Tip me back and carry me as far as the car: that's the easiest way on both of us, the doctor says. Then you're to drive me to the hospital, and they'll give me some oxygen."

Muriel stayed calm and relaxed while the men hoisted her down the steps.

'I'll make an apple pie for you when I get back," she said between heaving breaths. "But right now I'm supposed to keep still."

She did a good job of it. Ten days later, she was back to a full program, and able to make that apple pie.

Rescue squad. In most cities, the fastest way to get oxygen for a smothering type heart attack if you can't get to a hospital is through the rescue squad. Fire department equipment always includes oxygen, and workers are trained in its prompt use. Although some ambulances carry excellent oxygen equipment, others have nothing whatsoever to offer. Rescue squads usually are radio dispatched, too. And their services usually are free. If the situation seems desperate or your doctor cannot be reached, the rescue squad may be your best bet.

HOW TO HELP YOUR DOCTOR GET THE JUMP ON
HEART AND ARTERY TROUBLE

Your doctor can offer worthwhile help for many heart and artery troubles, but he can't do anything until you decide that something might be wrong and visit him. On the other hand, undue alarm at every twinge of chest pain keeps many people miserable and broke. How can you spot the conditions which your doctor can help without undue alarm or expense?

Heart complaints don't mean heart trouble even half the time. Here's one cheerful fact: if you go to your doctor because you think you might have heart disease, the odds are overwhelming that your heart will be all right! Here's a list of complaints which often send patients into a tailspin of worry and concern, when actually they seldom mean heart trouble or any serious bodily disease at all:

> Pain under the left nipple or low in the left chest.
> Palpitations or pounding of the heart.
> A smothering sensation with deep and slow breathing.
> Light-headedness with numbness of the hands and feet.

Even real heart failure can be stopped before it starts. Most people think that the heart beats faster and harder when it gets over-burdened, and then suddenly quits. They've had plenty of chance to soak up this false and terrifying idea, from the very words "heart failure" to well-meant but scare-type propaganda.

Don't let left-overs from such old-fashioned nonsense frighten you! If your heart ever finds itself under strain, it'll give you plenty of warning. You'll have time to get help, and the help you get will stand you in good stead.

Twinges of heart misery give valuable warning. Brief heart discomfort may give enough warning to let your doctor ward off an impending coronary heart attack for you. Such heart misery comes on abruptly. It usually strikes with overload from heavy activity, strong emotion, or extra eating. The pain is in the middle of the chest, and seems to cut off your breath. One patient called it "a fist shoving into my chest"—not a cramp, a searing pain or knife-like twinges, but a feeling of world-crushing weight. Discomfort may spread up to the neck or down either arm. One tip-off is that the victim instinctively sits or lies down and stays quite still during an attack instead of restlessly rolling or moving about. Don't confuse such pain with mere indigestion. Attacks like this, even though they pass off in a few minutes, means that a doctor's care can help you a great deal.

Sluggish heart action. Sluggish heart action or leaking valve trouble gives its first warnings through swollen feet and congested lungs. When the heart doesn't pump blood freely from the veins, pressure backs up to the tiniest, least water-tight vessels. The blood juices leak out. When you are up, the weight of the blood makes extra congestion in the feet and ankles. Swelling occurs there. At night, this swelling leaves. With the whole body level, fluid pools in the spongy lungs, which become water-logged and inefficient.

That's the background for the early signs of sluggish heart action, namely:

Evening swelling of the feet and ankles. When you notice this sign, press your finger firmly on the swollen area for ten seconds. If it leaves a definite dent, see your doctor the next day, even though the swelling has disappeared by then.

Too quick loss of wind with exertion. Breathing is rapid and shallow, with the chest partly full all the time. Things you could ordinarily do without trouble, like walking up one flight of stairs or working at a normal rate, make you lose your wind.

Loss of wind in the middle of the night. Patients often tell how they get up in the middle of the night because the room seems stuffy. A few minutes' sitting by the open window relieves them. But it isn't really the open window that helps: it's sitting up so that the fluid siphons downhill out of the lungs to other body parts. If such a spell hits you with the rapid, shallow breathing of true heart trouble, prop yourself up on three or four pillows or in an easy chair. If the attack doesn't subside, get help. If it does, go see your doctor in the morning to avoid further difficulty.

Rheumatic fever. Don't you get a wonderful feeling of relief when your doctor tells you that there is no leak in any of your heart valves? You can enjoy that feeling through the years, thanks to a new advance in medicine. Most leaky valves come from rheumatic fever, and rheumatic fever now can be held off by killing the family of germs that triggers each attack.

Penicillin or sulfa. The American Heart Association gives penicillin top billing for rheumatic fever control. One or two tablets a day almost always prevents the heart-crippling form of rheumatism. Sulfa derivatives fill in for patients who can't take penicillin. You should check with your doctor about this technique if you've ever had rheumatic fever, inflammatory rheumatism, or a rheumatic-type heart murmur. Under these conditions, one visit to your doctor and one or two pills a day will practically eliminate your extra risk of valve leakage.

HOME CARE CAN BANISH MANY INNOCENT
CHEST PAINS

Proper home measures cure almost all of the pains and twinges in the chest and upper abdomen which cause people concern and discomfort without actually being due to heart or lung disease. Probably the commonest such condition is *pinched nerve chest pain*, which causes steady, dull discomfort or sudden twinges along one or more rib segments. This condition usually strikes after you have been sitting in a cramped position for several hours: driving a car, working at a desk with one arm hanging unsupported from your shoulder or the like. The weight of your shoulder and arm pushing down on your ribs lets the muscles between the ribs pinch tender nerves. The pinched nerves make these muscles cramp tight, causing still more damage. The next day you suffer from pain in one side of your chest, most often on the left but sometimes on the right or on both sides. You can get relief from pinched nerve chest pain by this simple exercise:

Chest stretching. Sit sidewise in a tough chair, preferably with a back high enough that its top falls just opposite your nipple, with your left side toward the chair back. If the chair back is too tall, sit on a telephone book or cushion. Let your left arm hang behind the chair so that your ribs are against the chair back. Reach your right arm straight up toward the ceiling. Bend your right elbow and put the fingertips of your right hand on your left ear. Now bend your body across the chair back, tipping your right elbow as far as possible toward the left and stretching it up toward the ceiling. Let the chair back press against your left chest to act as a fulcrum. You should feel your right ribs spreading apart. Stretch the rib muscles in this way for three seconds. Switch to the other side and follow the same procedure. Stretch each side three times. Follow the whole routine three times a day until pain ceases. Ward off further discomfort by stretching exercises once a day thereafter.

Gas pains sometimes strike high enough in the chest to cause considerable confusion, too. The highest portion of your stomach, in which gas frequently accumulates, tents up underneath your diaphragm nearly to nipple level. Gas pains are generally on the left side instead of underneath the breastbone. They do not run down the arm as heart pain often does. Attacks sometimes follow over-eating or unusually rich food. A dose of bicarbonate and a carminative enema (see pages 51-52) often gives quick relief.

HOW TO FEND OFF HARDENING OF THE ARTERIES

Free blood flow through supple arteries keeps all your organs supplied with fuel and gives blood clots no harmful place to form.

The conditions that cut short the lives of nearly half of all Americans cannot strike. The decline people blame on old age will not visit you: enough moving blood keeps your memory sharp, your skin young, and your muscles strong.

Hardening of the arteries is a controllable disease. Hardening of the arteries comes from a scaly deposit in the wall of the blood vessels which carry blood to the tissues. This scaly deposit is made largely of cholesterol, a substance found in food, and also formed within your body during digestion of the fat that you eat. Hardening chokes off blood flow and makes rough places on which blood can clot. Clogged circulation means decline, which is what people fear about "old age." But the trouble isn't age! Hardening of the arteries is a disease that science can now prevent and even cure.

Why cholesterol forms scales within artery walls. Although nobody can prove exactly what chemical steps take place in depositing cholesterol within the wall of an artery, certain general principles seem established. Cholesterol and its chemical cousins form in vast quantities within your body when you eat certain fats. None of these substances dissolves freely in the blood or tissue fluids. Your body floats them through the circulation on protein rafts—giant molecules with soap-like ability to keep fatty substances suspended in water or blood. As tissue fluids filter through the artery wall to nourish it, some of these protein rafts get stuck. They are small enough to pass through the artery's inner lining, but too large to move all the way through the vessel wall. Chemical processes ultimately break down the trapped protein raft, leaving its cholesterol-molecule passenger stranded within the artery wall. The thickening and abnormal character of the vessel caused by the presence of cholesterol soon makes passage of other protein rafts still more difficult, leading to more and more stranded molecules, like traffic backed up from a single road-blocking stalled car during a Minnesota blizzard.

Attacks on the artery-hardening mechanism. Several links in this disease-forming chain are now being subjected to research attack. New soap-like substances have been found which carry the cholesterol on through artery walls, but unfortunately have proved to have undesirable poisonous qualities. The difference in protein rafts, only a small proportion of which are large enough to get stuck in their passage through the vessels, has been studied very intensely. Several substances have been found which greatly alter the size and shape of these rafts. One such substance is heparin, which unfortunately has profound effect on blood clotting and may lead to deadly hemorrhage unless dosage is rigidly controlled. Another such substance is made by the body in response to heparin and seems safe and effective, but cannot yet be manufactured. Perhaps new discoveries at any time will spell the end of hard arteries' deadly toll and prolong life for half of all Americans. Meanwhile, we can only control this condition by dietary and living methods. These have been conclusively proved to slow or reverse the hardening process, but only when applied day by day over a period of many years.

The fat you eat determines the cholesterol in your blood. Even though you eat considerable cholesterol in such foods as eggs, butter, and cream, dietary cholesterol makes little difference to your blood cholesterol level. The acids and enzymes in your stomach and intestine destroy much of the cholesterol in your food before it even soaks into your system. Cholesterol formed inside your body, from fats which you eat, really constitutes the bulk of the cholesterol in your blood at all times. Unless your body uses fats in an abnormal way, your program for lastingly supple arteries need not include any restriction on cholesterol-containing foods, which are tasty and easily obtained. Only a few people have abnormal cholesterol blood tests and need to follow a strict doctor-prescribed diet.

On the other hand, the amount and type of fat you eat very definitely affects your blood cholesterol content and therefore the rate at which your arteries become hard. Polyunsaturated fats, which tend to be liquid at room temperature, do much less harm than saturated fats, which tend to be solid. There is no doubt that your arteries will last longer and stay more supple if you eliminate as much saturated fat as you can practically do without, both by substituting liquid for solid fats and by limiting total fat intake.

You can find on any grocer's shelf the foods you need for keeping your arteries much more supple. You would have to give up many good foods if you wanted to go all out for supple arteries. But you can cut hardening of your arteries in half by choosing delicious, satisfying foods from your grocer's shelves. You can do this with no extra food costs at all, because no special foods are required. Just follow these three rules to keep supple, long-lasting arteries and younger tissues through the years:

1. Keep down the amount of harmful fat you eat with your meat. Eat harmless (or possibly helpful) veal, fish, or poultry twice a week. Trim off all visible fat from all types of meat. Avoid fat meats like bacon and fried or panbroiled meat, which has soaked up extra fat during preparation. Choose "economy" or "good" grade beef and pork instead of fatter "choice" or "prime."

2. Use liquid cooking oils in preference to solid shortenings whenever possible. Fat added for seasoning or as an ingredient and fat which soaks up into food during frying make up a large proportion of the fat you eat. Natural vegetable oils are not only harmless to your arteries but also help to cancel out the deleterious action of animal fats. The chemical processes ordinarily used to make such oils into solid shortenings convert them into the type of fat most researchers now feel is most harmful so you should use the oils in their natural, liquid form.

3. Keep the total fuel value of your foods down to the level which will support your body at its ideal weight. The absolute amount of undesirable fat you eat is what counts the most. Even if you follow the above rules, you will get at least 25 to 30 per cent of your calories from fat. (The American average is 42 per cent.) At least half of that fat will be of the undesirable animal or solidified variety. (The American average is 85 per cent.) You can eat enough of such food to sustain you at normal weight without worrying about your arteries. If you eat half again as much, your total intake of undesirable fat is nearly back where it started. A program to cut your weight back to its ideal level and keep it there is often practical (see Chapter Twelve), while more stringent limitation in proportion and type of fat is absolutely impossible without laboratory-prepared foods. That is why weight control is a key step in gaining full artery-sparing effect.

An artery-preserving diet is tasty, varied, and easy to follow. You can spare your arteries without depriving yourself of the pleasures of a well-set table. For example, look at the slight modifications one of my patients had to make when he took up this program. In the left column is the menu he would have followed ordinarily. Next is his new menu. Last an explanation of the changes involved.

ORDINARY:	ARTERY-SPARING:	CHANGES:
Breakfast:		
Grapefruit	Grapefruit	Omits fatty meat (ba-
Fried eggs and bacon	Eggs fried in vegetable	con) and uses vege-
Toast	oil	table oil instead of
Coffee	Toast	animal fat for fry-
	Coffee	ing
Lunch:		
Roast beef sandwich	Chicken sandwich	Substitutes chicken
Tossed salad with	Salad (same)	for beef, since he
French dressing	Apple pie (crust made	has no strong pre-

ORDINARY:	ARTERY-SPARING:	CHANGES:
Apple pie (crust made with solid shortening)	with vegetable oil) Milk	ference and poultry fat is less harmful than beef fat Makes crust with oil

Dinner:

ORDINARY:	ARTERY-SPARING:	CHANGES:
Panbroiled sirloin steak	Broiled sirloin steak	Steak broiled so that fat drips off instead of soaking back up into the meat
Baked potato	Baked potato	
Peas	Peas	
Lettuce and tomato salad	Lettuce and tomato salad	Peas not seasoned with butter or oleo in the kitchen
Chocolate cake	Chocolate cake	Cake and icing made with vegetable oil instead of solid shortening

If this patient had been a bit overweight, he might have made further changes. Boiled or poached eggs instead of fried, fresh fruit instead of pie, low calorie salad dressing or vinegar, and a low calorie pudding like D-Zerta instead of chocolate cake would knock perhaps six hundred calories off his day's total. After his weight was down, though, he could switch to a program like the one listed, which places very little strain on either the cook or the consumer.

Readers who wish to follow a somewhat more rigid artery-sparing diet because of past difficulty with hardening of the arteries, coronary heart attacks, or stroke, or because of a strong family tendency toward such illnesses, will find helpful directions and recipes in *The Low Fat Way to Health and Longer Life* (Prentice-Hall, Inc.), by Lester M. Morrison, M.D., and in *Eat Well and Stay Well* (Doubleday and Company), by Ancel and Margaret Keys.

Even easy artery-sparing diets may soon be unnecessary. If you eat out at restaurants or have poor control of how your food is prepared for other reasons, there's a bright ray on the horizon for you: close chemical cousins of cholesterol, called sitosterols, can be used to block the pathways which artery clogging substances take into your bloodstream from the intestine. The effect on your body when you take sitosterols as medicine is the same as if you stuck to a very low fat diet, and more—some additional cholesterol may be flushed out of your body. At the moment, this treatment is quite costly. The

time may soon come when we can enjoy lots of rich or fried food
and supple arteries, too, without prohibitive expense.

HOW TO AVOID CORONARY HEART TROUBLE

**When you avoid hardening of the arteries, you'll avoid coronary
heart attacks, too.** A great many heart attacks are due to stopping up
of one of the arteries through which the heart muscle itself gets fuel.
A clot is what stops up the artery, but clots only form after
hardening has made the vessel narrow and rough-walled. If you
follow the dietary measures we've discussed to keep your arteries
supple, you'll help your heart dodge most coronary attacks.

Two other measures give you further help:

1. You can open up your coronary arteries with muscular activity.
Daily, mild muscular activity opens your coronary arteries. This
makes coronary heart attacks less common and less severe. British
mailmen, for example, walk several miles each day. They have fewer
heart attacks than postal clerks with similar salary and status. The
few mail carriers who have heart attacks get much milder ones than
the clerks suffer. People who do heavy work have only one-third as
many heart attacks as people who do light work according to Drs.
Jeremy N. Morriss and Margaret D. Crawford of Britain's Medical
Research Council. In this country, nationally known authorities like
Dr. Paul D. White have long recommended regular exercise for every
reasonably healthy man or woman, regardless of age. All of these top
doctors agree that steady activity helps both by opening up existing
coronary blood vessels and by making extra detour channels develop,
so that the plugged coronary arteries which underlie most heart
attacks become less likely and less harmful.

Exercise. You can put yourself in the nearly-heart-attack-free class
by gradually building up your own activity unless you have severe
disease-imposed limitations. This activity ought to be regular and
mild. Most people find that walking a mile or two daily, riding a
bicycle to and from work, spending an hour in the garden or at the
bowling alley, or any of a dozen other interesting, useful pursuits will
fill the bill. The important things are these:

1. Pick something you can do daily.
2. Use heavy leg and trunk muscles mainly: then you can exert enough
effort to stimulate your heart without tiring yourself out.
3. Have a special activity planned for bad weather, off seasons, and times
when your schedule gets crowded.

Why not set up a program right now? Write down what you want to do, including second-bests. Decide right now to bowl twice a week if you can and to take a walk after supper whenever you can't. Or decide to spend an hour in either your garden or your workshop every day. Barring doctor's orders to the contrary, keep up this custom until you're 90 or more.

2. You can develop wholesome outlets for pent-up emotion. You have seen for yourself what strong emotions can do to human blood vessels. The pale face of fear, the flushed face of anger—almost all emotions involve violent and visible shifts in the size of surface blood vessels. Exactly the same changes occur in your inner organs. Different arteries clamp down during some strong emotions, engorge themselves during others. When vital arteries clamp down, blood flow in them slows, especially near the scale-narrowed spots in hardened arteries. If severe slowing occurs throughout your body, your blood pressure soars. If severe slowing strikes in the coronary vessels, a clot may form and cause a heart attack. Likewise with many other parts of the body: stopped blood vessels can cause stroke, sudden blindness, gangrene, and so on.

Such trouble develops mainly when tightness of the arteries continues for hours. Since emotion-induced tightness disappears when you express your feelings, ordinary emotions do no harm. Your blood pressure may soar when you're angry, but it drops quickly when you've said your piece. Only pent-up emotion creates lasting strain. Wholesome outlets for your feelings completely protect your body from most harmful effects of emotion.

What wholesome outlets? Three main ones are worthwhile.

A. Express your feelings freely whenever possible. You need considerable self-control. However, self-release is safe and useful, too. Some matters aggravate you, but aren't big enough to merit self-control. Some differences involve people who love you enough that they'll forgive a minor flare. In such circumstances, why not practice self-release on purpose, as you now practice self-control?

One of my coronary patients seemed quite meek. He never blew his top at anyone. Yet he was always inwardly upset. He boiled for hours after his wife called him "Baldy." He got mad as hops when his teenager took the family car without asking permission.

"Why don't you ever sound off?" I asked. "Tell them how you feel. You'll feel better, and they'll try not to annoy you quite as much."

"Maybe you're right, but I've never said a word before. I don't know how my family will react."

"You'll never know until you try. Just speak up right away whenever you're annoyed, in your own home. That'll be safe enough, I promise."

He tried blowing off steam with his own family. By the end of the month his heart condition was much improved, and so was his disposition.

"I'm doing the same thing at the office now," he told me. "I used to be afraid to say how I feel for fear people wouldn't like it. But they seem to like me better when they know just where they stand."

That's what he liked about his new behavior. But what I liked was something different: the pills he used for heart pain were all still in the bottle. He hadn't needed a single one. If too much self-control keeps you constantly constrained, and if your family's feelings can stand up under a little temporary upheaval, you will probably find similar release worthwhile.

B. Discuss and air your feelings. When you tell someone what has happened to you, you live the events over again in your mind. Can't you use this fact to set your feelings straight? To gain release and sympathy, and perhaps the satisfaction of saying all the things you wish you could have said, but didn't at the time?

One of my patients always used my offices this way, with my wholehearted consent.

"There's no one else I can talk to," he said one day. "My family's wound up in this, and my friends all gossip."

"Tell me about it," I said.

"It's my wife. She's always siding with my daughter Rose. The girl's getting sort of wild. Last night, I told her she'd have to stay home for a week, she'd been late so often. But my wife just told her to go on out with her boyfriend."

"I guess that made you mad, all right."

"Mad? I just couldn't open my mouth for fear of what I'd say. The others went on out to do the dishes—this happened right at supper—and I picked up the paper, but I couldn't read. I was in a perfect stew. I should have stormed right in there and told them a thing or two, that's what I should have done."

Does this conversation sound futile to you? It wasn't really. In the end, my patient calmed down and made up his mind to make the best of his home situation. He felt much better for going over his upheaval with me, even though it didn't really change things.

Perhaps you'll find some problems you can discuss with your close friends, your family, or your religious adviser. Perhaps you'll find it helpful to write letters, even if you never send them through the mails. Air your feelings! It's a real help, both to your mind and your body.

C. You can take out strong feeling on a substitute. One way to rid your body of pent-up feeling is to take it out on someone or something else. This certainly is bad at times: I don't advise anyone to beat his wife if he's had trouble with his boss, or kick his horse when his in-laws make him mad. But there are some substitutes that work perfectly well without making trouble or stirring later pangs of conscience. You can chop logs. You can hit golf balls. You can shoot rabbits. Such violent actions help to blow off steam without troubling your conscience or disturbing your life with your neighbors.

Do you need such release for yourself? Here's a brief self-quiz that will help you to decide. Answer these questions yes or no:

1. When someone has said something unpleasant or unfair, do you often think of a good retort when it's too late?
2. Do you feel abused sometimes?
3. Are you extremely proud of your self-control?
4. Are you frequently frustrated?
5. Do you feel wound up and tense for several hours after a disagreement?
6. Have you had high blood pressure or spells of heart pain?

If you answered "yes" to two or more questions, you definitely need a way of blowing off steam regularly. One "yes" means you could use such release at times, but needn't work it into your daily program. In either case, pick an appealing method from the list below, or choose something similar that suits your own needs. All

Safe Ways to Vent Your Spleen

Participation Sports:
Golf
Bowling
Darts
Hunting
Archery
Marksmanship

Spectator Sports:
Watching football
Watching wrestling
Watching hockey
Watching boxing

Hobbies and Crafts:
Whittling
Woodworking
Coppercraft or metalcraft
Sewing (in part)
Leather tooling
Gardening

Household Tasks:
Carpentry
Scrubbing floors
Hand washing
Chopping wood
Parts of cookery, such as pounding meats, mixing batters, chopping nuts

these things let you attack something physically, or give you the feeling of being in on such an effort. They're all entirely proper.

You can meet some resentments specifically. If there's one obvious thorn in your side, you can take even more specific steps to make it painless. Take the case of a union chief and how he handled this problem, for instance:

"You say I should let loose," he told me. "But I sit at the bargaining table with those slick-smiling goons, and I've got to smile, too. They're cutting the heart out of my plans, and they hate my guts. But I've got to work with them. It's my job to coop up my feelings."

"At the time, yes," I said. "But what about later?"

"When? After I quit this job?"

"No, each day. I'm going to have you paste their pictures on the wall down in your basement. I want you to throw darts at those guys. Score it however you please—ten points for an eye, five for a nose and two for an ear. Play with someone or all by yourself. But put in fifteen minutes at it every night."

Sound foolish? Maybe so. But it worked. My patient felt great relief. If someone constantly pushes you around and you can't talk back to him try one of these prescriptions: Throw darts at his picture. Paint his likeness on your chopping block. Picture him in your mind's eye as you take aim at a target with rifle, shotgun or bow. Think of his nice round head when you wallop a golf ball. You'll feel the pent-up anger flow from you as you carry out these plans.

HOW TO KEEP YOUR BLOOD PRESSURE DOWN

What makes blood pressure high? The arteries through which the blood flows become narrow, then the heart has to push extra hard to force blood through. The narrowed or tense arteries come first. The pounding, over-active heart comes later, if at all.

The measures we've discussed for keeping arteries supple help to hold your blood pressure down. Wholesome outlets for emotions also help: they relax all the arteries in your whole body and lower your blood pressure. These measures are extremely important, but there are also several specific ways to fight off high blood pressure.

Hold your blood pressure down by dodging excess salt. African tribes without ready access to salt don't suffer the scourge of high blood pressure. People who never salt their food or salt only to taste are less likely to have high blood pressure than those who salt their food without tasting it first. Although this has never been proved to be a cause and effect relationship, it seems reasonable to skip excess salt.

You can hold your blood pressure down through self-assertion. Like strong feelings, strong urges need outlets. When your just impulses are curbed, your blood pressure soars. Most experts say four out of every five cases of high blood pressure stem from such stresses rather than age, physical disease or strain. It's a dangerous tendency you can spot in yourself, as a frequently occurring frustrated, overtight, hurt feeling.

What can you do instead of fume inwardly? You can get in the habit of asserting yourself. Be decisive, definite, and prompt in every issue that is really up to you. That's how my patient, Jim Meadows, straightened himself out.

"People walk all over me," Jim said on his first visit. "My wife, my kids—everybody."

A three-point program changed all that:

First, Jim trained himself to make decisions promptly in areas where no one would argue. He made up his mind right away about what to wear, what to eat, and what to do.

Second, he learned to express himself promptly and definitely. He got rid of such phrases as "I think I'll have thus-and-so" and "maybe such-and-such would be all right for me." Instead, he said "I'll take thus-and-so" or "give me some of that, please."

Third, he said what he thought about contestable issues *before* the other fellow spoke up or took action. He trained himself to speak up quickly, without worrying about what the other fellow might think, whenever he was responsible for ultimate decision.

At the end of a month, Jim told me:

"I'm on the right track."

"Why, what's happened?" I asked.

"My wife asked me what I wanted to do last weekend instead of just making plans. First time since we've been married."

"Did you have your suggestions ready?"

"Well, not this time. But next time I will."

I'm sure he did. Jim didn't remake himself entirely—nobody ever does, or ever has to—but he made himself a power to be considered in his own home. In the process, he lost his feeling of pent-up containment and relieved his extra proneness to high blood pressure.

You may help your high blood pressure by getting reassurance. The actual facts about blood pressure aren't as bad as most people think. If your blood pressure has sometimes tested high, you can take comfort from these facts:

Moments of emotional upset won't cause a stroke no matter how high your blood pressure goes. Tests of the strength of brain arteries show that the highest pressures researchers could produce, more than five times the peak to which blood pressure rises in the worst cases of hypertension, do not blow out normal arteries. So forget the frightening notion that a stroke will punish you for slight anger if your blood pressure's up.

High blood pressure does not move inevitably toward higher pressure, heart failure or stroke, and death. Most patients with blood-pressure readings above normal either revert to normal at later rechecks or keep a safe, if slightly elevated, pressure for life.

You're not better or worse according to your exact blood pressure reading. It's the condition of your kidneys, blood vessels, and heart that really determines whether high blood pressure will cause you trouble. If your doctor can reassure you on these points, that means a lot more than the level of your blood pressure itself. Don't worry about exact numbers—they don't mean a thing.

CHAPTER FIFTEEN

How to Meet and Conquer Tumor Threats

"Cancer Death Rate Cut in Half!"

That's a headline everyone on earth would love to read. Yet it could be written today as far as you and your family are concerned. If you put present day knowledge of cancer to work, you can cut cancer's probable toll at least in half. You can prevent many cancers entirely. You can get complete, lifelong cure twice as often as the present average if cancer strikes. Even if the disease gets too far along for complete cure, you can often win a years-long reprieve while research bores closer to the ultimate cancer cure.

You can avoid many cancers altogether. The most hopeful word in the cancer field is this: as many as nine out of ten cancers of certain types, including several of the most common, can be avoided entirely! That doesn't mean merely that a painful, expensive operation can keep the victims out of the grave. It means that nine out of ten who would have had these forms of cancer can keep themselves from ever having an unhealthy day or needing a single treatment.

How can this be? Because science has proved that one big factor in starting many cancers is irritation. There are other factors, too—family tendencies, hormones, cosmic rays, and probably a dozen more that haven't been discovered yet—but the straw that breaks the camel's back is irritation. Avoid cancer-spurring irritation and you'll very probably avoid many varieties of cancer.

Irritation spurs cancerous growth. Bits of tissue are growing continually in your body. But they grow only to replace worn-out or injured bits nearby. The difference between normal tissue, simple tumors or growths, and cancerous growths is simply a matter of degree. All tissue grows. Tumor tissue grows more than it should, and presses on surrounding parts. Cancer tissue grows so violently that it can eat into normal tissue as well as press upon it.

Irritation definitely affects cellular growth. Anything which continually injures tiny bits of tissue so that they have to be replaced spurs more growth than would otherwise be needed. This increase in the rate of tissue growth sometimes spurs the exaggerated growth of cancer.

HOME MEASURES TO EASE CANCER-SPURRING IRRITATION

If you set out to dodge cancer-spurring irritation, a great deal of what you can do requires no medical aid or expense whatever. Here are three big steps:

1. Shield yourself from cancer-causing ultraviolet rays. Farmers and sailors get eight times as many cancers of the skin as indoor workers. The reason: excess sun exposure, with damaging amounts of ultraviolet light. Only the areas of skin exposed over a period of many years become increasingly cancer-bearing—the face, neck, and hands.

You can dodge excess ultraviolet rays without staying indoors or otherwise inconveniencing yourself. Don't worry about brief, in and out sun exposure. If you will be in the sun continuously for an hour or more, a broad-brimmed hat helps protect your face. A bit of unmedicated yellow petroleum jelly (Vaseline) will protect the backs of your hands or other heavily exposed areas for six to eight hours. A good suntan oil or cream will screen out most ultraviolet light, too. A preparation called "Uval" blocks almost all ultraviolet, if you need total protection.

2. You can protect your lungs against dangerous fumes and irritants. Scientists have actually found cancer causing irritants in the exhaust fumes of automobiles and trucks. The dangerous fumes are heavier than air. In heavy traffic, you should let fresh air into your car through the windows instead of using bumper-level ventilating ducts. You should also keep your car's exhaust system in good repair so you won't breathe in lung irritants from your own engine.

What about tobacco? Years ago, I used to shrug my shoulders at the quit-smoking crusades. My own consumption was over two packs of cigarettes a day. Then the facts began to pile up incontrovertibly.

What facts?

First, cancer of the lung was proved much more common in heavy smokers. Men who smoked as much as I were 52 times as likely to get cancer of the lung as nonsmokers. Even lighter smokers had a substantial extra tumor risk—pack-a-day men ran 22 times the nonsmoker rate, and half-a-pack-or-less men ran 11 times the non-smoker rate. Counting only the squamous cell cancers, the type tobacco-tar irritation seems to produce, the effect was even greater.

Second, cancer of the lung is a very common killer, especially among men. Actually, it is vying for first place.

Third, heavy cigarette smoking increases the chance of getting all kinds of cancer by two and a half times. It isn't just cancer of the lung—some still-unknown factor connects heavy cigarette smoking with cancer of the stomach, the bowel, the blood, and so forth.

Fourth, cancer-causing irritants have actually been found in cigarette-smoke residues. Animals get cancer after applications of certain concentrated cigarette-smoke tars.

Fifth, studies proved that the lung-lining cells reveal progressively more growth and more precancerous change the longer you smoke. A good lung pathologist can classify how close your lungs have moved to the cancer bearing state, and this judgment coincides closely with your past cigarette smoking habits.

Sixth, no known means of protection removes the risks from continued smoking. Filter tips, denicotined tobacco and so on seem thoroughly worthless. Switching to cigars cuts risk appreciably, but doesn't eliminate it entirely.

Seventh, less cancer isn't the only health benefit to be gained by discontinuing use of tobacco. Smokers of any type have more heart attacks and blood vessel disorders. Smoking hasn't been proved responsible, but if even half the heavy smoker's extra heart and blood vessel troubles are due to the tobacco itself, conquering the habit will add years to his life. Emphysema and several other lung conditions also punish many smokers for a few too many "puffs."

When I added up the totals in my own case, I found that smoking was slated to cost me at least ten years of life span. I figured it was worth a little discomfort to gain that much time on earth. So I quit smoking.

HOW TO QUIT SMOKING IF YOU DECIDE THAT'S BEST

You might get enough satisfaction from tobacco to make it worth the years it costs you. You might want to switch to cigars or a pipe. But if you want to quit smoking, there is one way to make it easier on yourself.

Smokers have a different breathing rhythm from non-smokers. A non-smoker breathes constantly at a rate and depth which keeps his body supplied with oxygen and free of certain wastes. The smoker breathes slightly more heavily while smoking and for a few minutes thereafter, then gradually breathes less deeply and less rapidly. Soon he becomes uncomfortable and feels the need of a cigarette. But is it really the tobacco, or the extra blood-purification which will come with smoke-spurred breathing which he craves? An article in *The Journal of the American Medical Association* recently suggested the latter. As the article suggests, I've had my patients take breathing exercises, then quit smoking while continuing the breathing program. Most of them find that they cut tobacco craving substantially in this way.

What kind of breathing exercises? Left hand on the hip, right hand on the tummy, stand erect. Breathe in through your nose, at first without raising your chest. Only after the lung is as full of air as you can get it by moving the diaphragm, which pushes the tummy out under your hand, should the chest begin to rise. Fill the lungs completely, then breathe out slowly through your mouth. Do this ten times, and repeat the whole procedure three times a day. After three weeks, quit smoking but continue the excercises for at least three months. If tobacco craving strikes, take time out for extra breathing exercise. Use any other helpful measures you've found, like gum-chewing or eating extra crackers, along with the breathing method.

Breathing exercises really work. All but one of the patients who have reported back to me are enthusiastic about this program. Here's the most extreme case:

J.G. smiled ruefully when I told him he ought to quit smoking.

"Every doctor I've seen since I got my ulcer has said that," he said. "Believe me, I've tried! Like they say, 'Anybody can quit smoking: I've done it a hundred times.' "

"Let's try it once more," I said. "This time maybe we can make it stick."

J.G. listened with interest while I explained the breathing exercise method. Six months later, he was back for another checkup on his stomach.

"I'm off the weed at last," he told me. "That breathing business really works!"

If J.G. couldn't quit when ulcer pains punished every forbidden puff, I doubt if he ever could have made it without breathing exercises. With their help, he managed to quit at last.

3. You can avoid cancer-spurring irritation by cleansing intimate body parts. Men in the waterless deserts of the world, where bathing is seldom possible, have to choose between circumcision and a high rate of sex organ cancer. A cheesy oil forms under the normal foreskin. If it is left there, it causes irritation. Over the years, this increases the chance of cancer tremendously.

Proper cleansing lets you avoid this tumor risk easily without circumcision. Every uncircumcised man and boy should strip back the foreskin at least once a week during a bath and wash thoroughly, then replace the foreskin in its normal position.

If you're a woman, it's harder to prove that you'll benefit from special cleansing methods of the sex organs. Thorough bathing of the outer portions of the female organ is probably wise at least twice weekly. Douching and other more complex methods have never been proved to ward off cancer.

HOW TO HELP YOUR DOCTOR TO FIGHT CANCER-SPURRING IRRITATION

Your doctor can cure cancer-spurring states at the mouth of the womb. At Memorial Hospital, over a thousand women reported twice a year for ten years to have cancer checkups for their pelvic organs. Two cancers were found, both in an early, readily cured state. But the amazing thing was that there were only two: considering the age of the women studied, doctors had expected at least twenty malignant growths. Why hadn't the other eighteen occurred?

Going back over the records, they found that many of the women had been treated for infection at the mouth of the womb. This infection was of a type that starts by itself, without being spread by sex contact or dirtiness. Treatment for it is painless and cheap, but apparently keeps nine out of ten cancers from ever getting a start.

If you're a woman you can avoid nearly one-sixth of your whole cancer problem by stopping any cancer-spurring irritation at the mouth of your womb. Your doctor's number one job in cancer control is to check the mouth of your womb at least once a year and treat any infection he finds lingering there.

Your dentist can help you dodge cancer. Another important form of cancer-spurring irritation involves the tissue inside your mouth. These cells are often spurred into dangerous types of growth by the rubbing of your cheek or tongue against a harsh place on a tooth or the pressure of a poorly fitted denture or bridge. You get used to these things so that you hardly notice them. But you can easily steer away from big cancer risks by clearing up such states. A trip to your dentist whenever you notice irritating roughness or denture misfits will pay off in banished cancer risks, with the extra comfort a pure gift.

HOW TO IDENTIFY AND RID YOURSELF OF INNOCENT GROWTHS AND CANCER VANGUARDS

When benign growths or cancer vanguards strike, you can often take curative action for yourself. In other cases, you can assure yourself a quick, inexpensive, and more comfortable doctor-managed cure by spotting the problem and getting help promptly. Consider first the frequently self-cured, benign conditions:

Warts. If you have had a succession of ordinary or plantar warts or have suffered along with medically diagnosed warts because of lack of money or time to have them removed, home techniques may well be the answer.

Dichloracetic acid. Carefully apply a thick layer of petroleum jelly all around the wart so that every bit of normal skin is protected. Dip the tip of a toothpick in dichloracetic acid, obtainable at your drugstore without a prescription. Apply it carefully to the surface of the wart. Use just enough acid to moisten the wart surface. Let it soak in for one minute, then blot once with cotton to absorb excess acid. Clean off the jelly and cover with a small bandage. Repeat the application at three day intervals, trimming or scraping off dead-white destroyed tissue if necessary, until the entire wart and its roots have been destroyed.

Ganglion. A ganglion is a bulge in the lubricated sheath around your tendons. The commonest variety occurs on the back of your wrist, and pops up as a prominent, smooth bulge whenever you bend the wrist down sharply. Sometimes the wrist is a bit sore and weak, too.

How to pop a ganglion. The old fashioned cure for ganglions was a wallop with the family Bible, which scattered the fluid from them through the wrist tissues quite thoroughly. Unfortunately, people who use this method sometimes break their wrists if they wallop too hard. A much safer method which works equally well on a thin-walled ganglion is to press down on the top of the knuckles with the heel of your other hand and bend the wrist sharply, then pinch the ganglion very firmly and steadily between thumb and forefinger. Sometimes you cannot make enough pressure yourself to burst the bubble, but one of your relatives can break the bulge between the pulps of his two thumbs.

A ganglion treated in this way may come back, but surgery is no more difficult than it would have been if you had never tried for a home cure.

Skin tags. Many people have tags which hang like tiny punching bags from their normal skin. Such tags have smooth surfaces and normal skin texture. Skin tags are harmless, but sometimes are so located that they frequently become irritated by the pressure of clothing. Your doctor can spark these off almost painlessly with an electric needle, to cure them. If you would rather go through a little discomfort than part with a surgeon's fee, though, one home technique is usually safe.

Ligature removal. If you tie a string tightly around the base of a skin tag, lack of blood will make it wither and die in a matter of seven to ten days. The string must be tight enough to stop up the arteries as well as the veins: otherwise the tag becomes extra swollen and sore. The best way to tighten the string is by winding the ends around your little fingers, making your hands into fists, and pressing your knuckles together like rockers. In this way, you will not rip the tag loose if the string happens to break while you are tightening it.

YOU CAN SPOT MANY CANCER VANGUARDS FOR YOURSELF

Three of the main types of cancer vanguards lie right on the surface of the body, where you can easily spot them for yourself. These conditions are not cancers. However, they are disturbances in cellular growth or stability which frequently allow cancer to start. Your doctor can remove or cure each of these conditions without risk or major expense, and usually without hospitalization or lost working time. Once a month, undress in a well-lit room and look for these signs:

1. Heaped-up skin cells. Some heaped-up skin cells form little horns, curving up to a noticeable point. Others are pearly-gray, dull, dry spots. The commonest ones are brownish, rough-edged spots. Whenever any of these types appear, get your doctor to take care of them. If you get many small spots, a freezing spray and quick scrape can make short, painless work of a dozen or more at a visit. If you get a few deeper spots, the electric needle or X-ray will cure them.

Rancher's skin. If you have thin skin, a pink-cheeked, dry complexion, and spend a lot of time in the wind and rain, you are especially likely to get heaped-up skin cells. Cut down the number of spots by washing your face and neck every day and rubbing-in lanolin skin cream.

2. White patches. Leather-like whitish patches on the lip, mouth, tongue, or female organ are also vanguards of cancer. These white patches most often come where there is some irritation from rough teeth, from a quid of chewing tobacco, or from a stream of hot pipe smoke. Whether you can see any reason for them or not, they are cancer vanguards and deserve a doctor's care.

3. Moles. Most moles are harmless. The few that might be dangerous are these:

1. Moles which you scrape when you shave.
2. Moles on your ankles or feet.
3. Moles which become irritated from the rubbing of clothing or underclothing.
4. Moles which change in size, shape, or color.

How Jim Moore got himself cured before cancer got a start. "I've got this scaly patch on my forehead," Jim told his doctor. "What is it?"

The spot was brownish, rougher than the skin around it, with craggy edges. It felt dry and harsh.

"It's from heaped up skin cells," the doctor said. "It's not a cancer. But if you leave it alone, there's a good chance it'll turn to cancer some day."

"Then I need an operation?"

"Not much of one. We'll inject something to keep it from hurting and burn off the spot with an electric needle. In about three weeks, the scab will drop off and you'll be well."

Ten minutes later, Jim Moore left the office. He was a few dollars poorer than when he went in, but had otherwise suffered no pain. Still, he'd rid himself of a real cancer threat.

HOW YOUR DOCTOR CAN HELP YOU FIND AND REMOVE TUMOR THREATS

Your doctor can find some cancer vanguards which you'd never see. Your doctor can get a good look at parts of your body which you can never see. He knows exactly what to look for. And he can find some cancer vanguards that aren't at the body surface, like growths in the ovaries, inside the bladder or in the large bowel. Whenever you see your doctor for other illness, why not ask him to look you over thoroughly for cancer vanguards, too?

Your doctor can cure many cancers completely. If cancer should strike in spite of everything you do to prevent it, your doctor still has better than a fifty-fifty chance of curing it for you completely.

But he can do nothing toward your cure until you take the first step by visiting his office.

When you make your monthly check for cancer vanguards, go through this checklist, too. None of the signs we'll list means that you absolutely have cancer. They only mean that you *might* have a tumor which deserves prompt care. You can double your chance of cure if cancer should strike by seeing your doctor whenever these signs cause suspicion:

1. A sore or spot that does not heal. People often first notice a growth when they bump against it or scrape it. A true cut or scrape should get well inside three weeks. After that time, it's worth checking with your doctor to see whether a tumor might be present.

Most of the time, a true tumor appears as a scab or bump. The scab may fall off or the center of the bump turn angry after a few days or weeks. The spot then looks like a tiny molehill completely surrounding a reddish dent. It usually isn't very sore or tender. Watch for such marks especially on the face, the back of the hands, the lip, tongue and mouth. See your doctor whenever one shows up: if it proves to be cancer, you'll have a better than 95 per cent chance of cure with prompt care.

2. A lump, bunch, or bulge. Take time out right now to find out how your skin and surface parts look and feel. There's probably some knobbiness about your finger joints. There may be clumps of birdshot-sized lumpiness in your breasts. Otherwise, your body should be smooth, and the two sides should more or less match.

When a growth forms on or near the surface of your body, you will be able either to see or to feel it. Skin growths look like tiny raised spots or scabs at first. They feel quite firm. Growths under the skin may show as bumps, but are easier to feel than to see. Growths far beneath the skin may show as a general bulging in the area above them, mainly notable when you compare the two sides. Strip completely in a well-lit room once a month to search for tumors. A shaving mirror with one side curved for extra magnification will help. Feel for lumps, too: you may find some with your fingers which you would miss with your eyes.

Breast examination. If you're a woman, you should check your breasts for lumps with special care. As long as menstrual periods continue, the best time of the month is immediately after bleeding stops. That's when normal gland tissue in the breast is softest and least likely to cause false alarms. After periods cease, make a point of feeling your breasts the first day of every month. Lie on your back with a small pillow or folded blanket under your right shoulder blade and with your right arm curled above your head. Lay your left hand on your right breast with the fingers close together and straight. Use the palm surface of the fingers instead of the tips, and feel by rubbing your hand in a gentle circle. You will catch any lumps against the smooth, solid backing of ribs and muscles. Cover each quarter of the breast in this way—upper outer, upper inner, lower inner, and lower outer. Then bring your right arm down from above your head to your side and repeat, being especially careful to cover the tag of breast tissue that reaches up toward the armpit. Change position and examine the other breast in the same way.

If you're like most women, you'll find two or three areas which don't feel quite right. There will be no real lump, but a sort of inner coarseness. This is normal breast tissue. After an interval, you will get to know how your breast should feel. After that, you'll spot a new lump or thickening with ease. And if you do spot one you'll have better than three out of four chances of lifelong cure even if it proves to be the worst possible kind of growth, as long as you see your doctor promptly.

Mary Rowen found a lump and lived. Mrs. Rowen sat on the very edge of her chair in my consulting room.

"I'd like you to check my breast, doctor," she said tensely.

Two days later, the lump Mary Rowen had found was in a laboratory bottle and Mary herself was getting well. She's stayed well for many years since, despite the fact that the lump was a cancer. She will stay well the rest of her life, thanks to the one minute a month she spent searching her breasts with her fingers.

3. Unusual bleeding. Here's where human nature does us a bad turn. Things seem to be back to normal inside a few minutes after hemorrhage. The natural thing to do is wait to see whether it happens again. The trouble is that bleeding which is due to early, curable cancer may not happen again for weeks or months. Most growths which cause bleeding offer an excellent chance for cure, but each week of waiting wastes part of that possibility. It's smart to watch for these particular forms of bleeding, and see your doctor the first time they show up:

1. Blood mixed with your urine.
2. Bloody bowel movement.
3. Black, tar-colored, soft, and bulky bowel movement, which may mean blood is being poured into the upper intestine and digested into tarry matter.
4. Bleeding, even involving only a few spots of blood, between menstrual periods or after the menopause. If such bleeding occurs after sexual relations,

don't ignore it on that account—that's when first bleeding occurs in many tumors.

5. Bloody or rusty looking material coughed up from the lungs, or severe, unexplained nosebleeds.

4. Unusual flux or discharge. A watery flow of matter from the female organs which makes the area itch or burn is sometimes due to a serious growth. There are also less serious causes, but this sign always calls for a doctor's examination.

5. Lasting stomach trouble. If you have stomach distress or difficulty swallowing several times a week for three weeks, it's time you talked to your doctor.

6. Change in your bowel habits. Nobody can tell how often you ought to empty your bowels. I've had normal patients who had a movement once in five days, and others who went three times a day or more. But whatever is right for you now ought to be right for you next month, too. If your bowels get suddenly tight or get very loose one week and very tight the next, if you get the feeling that you ought to go but find it impossible to get rid of anything but a little gas, or if you frequently pass little pencil-sized stools, see your doctor.

7. Change in your voice or altered cough. Hoarseness should clear up after two weeks or less. If it lasts longer, get medical attention. You'll win a cure about nine times in ten by prompt care, even if it's the worst thing it could be.

Cough is another matter. Almost everybody coughs up a little loose phlegm once in a while. You probably have to watch for change in your cough, not a brand-new cough. What kind of change? New brassiness, increased depth, accompanying chest pain, foul-smelling or bloody phlegm—any major change should have attention. Again, the odds are that an innocent cause will be found and quickly cured. But if something serious is present, you'll gain by prompt attention.

CHAPTER SIXTEEN

Home Remedies for
Family Planning

When the early settlers came to Minnesota, they actually *needed* children. It took more than four hands and more than two backs to break the foot-thick sod, to plant, to till, to harvest—and to get all of it done before the six-month winter. But even while they were still scratching for the barest living, our settlers looked out for their children's future. They put *education* next to *survival* on their lists, and built schools years before their first hospital.

To this day, we have a lot of carry-over from those times. Most people hereabouts want children, and also want to be sure that their children enjoy a life of opportunity and self-improvement. Usually this involves home or prescription remedies in two ways: to *increase* fertility when wanted pregnancies fail to occur, and to *decrease* it when family size or circumstances threaten to outrun the parents' ability to provide topnotch care and full opportunity.

WHEN YOU *WANT* CHILDREN

The term "family planning" has one bad feature: it gives you the idea that once you decide to have a child, nature will automatically cooperate. In actual fact, a couple who are fully fertile and capable of having a child may need a long time to get a pregnancy started. Such couples average 10 months of trying before conception occurs. I usually tell people who are worried about infertility to wait for at least two years before taking any special steps. Even then a fair number will go ahead and conceive before the tests are finished. So, ladies, don't fret if you can't get pregnant the first few months you try.

"Not fretting" may actually help to solve the problem. Every doctor has seen women who try harder and harder to get pregnant,

232

with more and more striving and straining and concern, and don't get anywhere. Finally they conclude that they will never have a natural child, go out and adopt a baby, quit straining to get pregnant, and conceive the next month. The anxiety and tension connected with striving can actually change the openness of one's tubes and other physical factors concerned in getting pregnant. If you can "let the chips fall where they may" in a relaxed way, pregnancy is actually more likely.

Still, you may need to take some special measures if you have trouble getting pregnant. Here are several suggestions.

Rhythm in reverse. Generally speaking, a woman only develops one egg cell a month to a state of full ripeness. This cell must be fertilized within three days or it passes on. The sperm which meet it can come from intercourse during the egg's three-day survival period, or can be in the birth passage up to two days ahead of time.

The most you ever have, then, is only five days of true fertility each month. The so-called rhythm method of birth control (aimed mainly at *preventing* rather than *promoting* pregnancy) adds two more days on each end of the fertile period for "safety," and defines the 9th to the 19th day (counting the day menstrual flow begins as day 1) as the fertile period. If you're trying to concentrate your efforts when they will do the most good, though, the 12th through the 16th day deserve the most attention. This assumes a 28-day cycle and "average" time of ovulation, which works out right for about two-thirds of women.

What about the others? If your cycle is longer or shorter than usual, your fertile time usually is correspondingly later or earlier. In other words, if your cycle is 31 days (3 days longer than average) your fertile time is the 15th through the 19th day, if 25 days (3 shorter) it is the 9th through the 13th day.

If you want to go all out for faster results, you can zero in on your most fertile moment by taking your temperature daily before you get up or stir around in the morning. Be sure to shake the thermometer all the way down, because your normal temperature under these conditions may be 97 degrees or less. Starting on the first day of menstruation, you will probably have low readings for several days. There may then be an unusually low reading for one day, followed by daily readings about half a degree higher than before. The "dip" may or may not show up, but the rise almost always does. Ovulation generally occurs at the time of the "dip" or the day before the rise to a new plateau. One couple who had tried for several years to have a child found that in spite of a normal cycle the wife's most fertile period centered on her fifth or sixth day. Since they had been following Orthodox Jewish rules (which prohibit intercourse during and for seven days after menstruation), she had really had no opportunity to get pregnant. Revamping the couple's sex schedule (with intercourse concentrated on the fourth through seventh days) solved their problem in a hurry, as the rather crowded family picture on my desk clearly reveals.

Acid-fighting douches. During most of the month, the vagina bathes its own walls with an acidic fluid. The acid keeps germs out of the birth passage, but also quickly kills off any sperm which encounter it. Acidity decreases sharply in most women just at the time of the month when they are most fertile, but many of the women who have come to me for help with infertility have had a high level of vaginal acidity throughout the cycle.

Theoretically, you could easily test yourself for this condition. Practically speaking, however, the cure is easier than the test. Just mix two teaspoonsful of baking soda (sodium bicarbonate) in 1 quart of lukewarm water and use as a douche, following the directions in Chapter 6 (p. 89). Douche according to these directions at bedtime, so that the douche will presumably precede intercourse by two hours or less, whenever you expect to have relations. If neutralizing vaginal acids is going to help, it will usually be effective within the first three months, but the program is harmless if you want to try it for a little longer.

Knee chest position. When a woman lies on her back, fluids within the vagina tend to flow toward the back of her vagina and down toward the outside. Since the sperm are only effective if they get up into the uterus, which communicates with the front surface of the vagina high inside, this flow reduces the chance of pregnancy. Particularly if you have used acid-fighting douches so that sperm which fail to enter the upper birth tract immediately can still survive, positions which allow sperm-carrying fluids to puddle in the upper front vagina often aid fertility. For fullest effect, intercourse should be performed with the wife kneeling on the bed with her chest either on the mattress or resting on one pillow. Her husband kneels behind her to perform intercourse. Following relations, the wife should lie on her stomach for half an hour. This same procedure also aids fertility in women with tipped uterus, since gravity tends to straighten out the birth passages.

I recently had a letter from a patient to whom I had recommended knee chest position. Her note came straight to the point: "It's a boy, and thanks!" I've never kept track of successes and failures, but I know that a number of couples who had tried other approaches for years have been able to have a family this way.

SOME CHILDREN BUT NOT TOO MANY

One trouble with the family planning notion is that it sounds so definite. Either you *want* children and you are straining to get pregnant or you *don't want* them and you are anxious, fearful and concerned. Either way, harmful emotions intrude upon your sex life, which generally proves most satisfying if you can approach intercourse in a framework of "whatever will be, will be." The effect often proves considerable, and may make a slight change in approach quite worthwhile.

The change amounts simply to accepting approximate rather than absolute control of family size, spacing and so forth. The "strict planning" approach makes you try hard to have a child during one period, then try just as hard not to have another for the next ten or fifteen years. Doesn't it make more sense simply to take mild measures to reduce fertility and accept the baby whenever it arrives? Just avoiding intercourse or using foam (see below) during the 9th to 19th days (counting the first day of menstruation as Day One) cuts fertility to an average of less than half. Following such a program from the start, even though you want children, will cut your family to very nearly the "usual" size without requiring more strenuous measures, and allows a fully receptive attitude whenever a pregnancy occurs.

NO PREGNANCIES, PLEASE!

Over half of our maiden beauties in Minnesota are married by the time they are twenty. If the fertile couples formed through these marriages took no steps whatever to limit reproduction, they would average about thirteen children each. (Figuring one conception every ten nonpregnant months, 75 per cent of the pregnancies surviving to live birth, 25 years to menopause.) So the question with regard to birth control isn't *if*, it is *how*.

ABSTINENCE

Despite its perfect efficiency and low dollar cost, simply omitting intercourse usually doesn't even receive honorable mention as a birth control measure. Yet I have seen a good many couples, particularly of the older generation, who controlled family spacing and size entirely by this means. If both man and wife view their sex life mainly as the means of reproduction rather than as a major reward of being married, or if they think of the family primarily as an economic team (which it still is on many Minnesota farms), this approach can work out well. Most couples today expect pleasure and fulfillment as well as reproduction from their sex life, and cannot refrain from intercourse year after year. Having seen the vast influence of a happy sex life on the whole family's emotional life, I have to agree that abstinence meets the needs of only a few, very special couples.

RHYTHM METHODS

You can cut the number of pregnancies approximately in half either by avoiding intercourse or by using sperm blocking methods (see below) during the most fertile ten days of the menstrual cycle. This makes sense if you are trying to produce "some but not too many" children, but it isn't good enough for single girls, women with health problems, or couples for whom a pregnancy would produce really tragic results.

Douches. Douching immediately after intercourse seems a common-sense measure to reduce fertility. Unfortunately, douching is just as likely to wash sperm up into the crucial zones as back away from them. Douching for this purpose is at best useless and at worst (with strong chemicals) harmful. I strongly advise against it.

Sperm barriers. Short of the pill, the most effective ways of avoiding pregnancy keep sperm out of the upper birth passage, where conception occurs. An actual physical barrier has adverse effects on couple sex life. A wall of rubber, whether condom, diaphragm or sheath, gives a distinct shower-in-a-raincoat effect. A chemical barrier interferes much less with normal sensation, and thus seems much more natural. Natural contact seems much more important than a chemical-free technique, especially since the chemicals involved do not soak into your system. So the barrier I recommend is vaginal foam, either Delfen or Emko brand, available without a prescription in most drugstores. Either brand comes with an applicator made up of a plastic tube and plunger. Pressing the container's tip into the plastic tube causes foam to push up the plunger and fill the applicator. You then insert this high into the vagina like a tampon, and push the plunger to deposit foam well inside. Although the directions say that one applicatorful is enough, I advise two applicatorsful when this is being used as the only means of birth control.

Preparation can be taken "just in case," in which event you will be protected for at least four hours, or immediately before intercourse. A fresh applicatorful should be applied if you have intercourse a second time during the same night, since secretions thin out the ingredients too much for multiple use.

Foams control conception about twice as well as the traditional devices, and interfere a great deal less with natural contact. They have absolutely no effect on your body's hormone balance and have never been related to cancer, vein clots or other serious disease. I have seen a couple of women who developed a temporary redness and itching from allergy to one or another ingredient and had to switch to another method, but no serious aftereffects at all. The only real problem is "mess" from leakage of material, which may in some instances justify use of a plastic-backed disposable bed pad or application of Kotex after intercourse.

Coils and loops. The uterus and tubes normally milk material within them gently toward the exterior, keeping dirt or bacteria from working up the birth passage. When a foreign object is inside, these milking movements become much stronger. In the process, any fluid or floating object is quickly cast forth. Since the egg cell normally floats gently down this passage toward where the sperm will meet it, increased movement generally casts the egg cell out before fertilization can occur.

A coil or loop within the uterus causes these increased movements constantly, and thus works rather effectively to prevent pregnancies. These devices do not cause abortion—if a pregnancy occurs, the developing baby simply crowds the loop or coil aside—but they do reduce conceptions to about one for each twenty years. And coils or loops are fairly natural in their action: they do not interfere in any way with marital contact or with your body's hormone balance.

There are two common drawbacks to this birth control method. The first is that a doctor has to put the loop or coil in place and check it periodically, which involves inconvenience and cost. The second is that some women either expel the device or get cramps, bleeding or other side effects from excessive milking movements in the uterus. After a pregnancy or two, most women get along fine with an intrauterine device. At the start of reproductive life, though, many must switch to a different method.

Pregnancy pretense pills. Never in the history of mankind have so many people taken such powerful medication for so long a period *when they were not even sick* as have taken birth control pills. The hormones required come very close to the total amounts which turn a young girl into a mature woman. Make no mistake: birth control pills involve major meddling with bodily and mental functioning.

On the other hand, this meddling did not create a new and unfamiliar state. Instead, it originally mimicked pregnancy, whose effects on various body systems have long been known. Once a woman is pregnant, her body stops forming egg cells. This keeps her from ever carrying twins of different ages, who would have no chance of normal birth. "The pill" triggers this mechanism by artificially matching the hormone status of pregnancy.

Women who take "the pill" regularly can depend almost 100 per cent on its efficiency. At the same time, they may suffer some of the discomfitures of a pregnancy, such as morning sickness, easy fatigue and weight gain. The effect on sex drive and interest varies sharply. Some women find release from pregnancy fears improves the physical side of marital relations. A few don't want their husbands to get anywhere near them. In this circumstance, I advise a switch to other methods—foam, loops or coils, or the cycle-confusing pill (discussed below).

How to prevent leg vein clots with the pill. We used to think that leg vein clots in pregnancy occurred because the growing uterus pressed on the veins through which blood had to return from the legs toward the heart. Then along came "the pill," and with it some increase in leg vein clots. The increase is not tremendous, but it certainly deserves attention.

Take Mildred's case, for instance. She came to me just after the leg vein problem had a big publicity splash.

"I really hate to give up the pill," she said. "It's been so wonderful to have a method we can really depend on, and without any mess or clutter. But this blood clot business has me really worried."

"I'm sure it has. But let's get a little more information before we decide what to do. What about your family history—have any of your relatives had strokes or heart attacks or other blood vessel conditions?"

"My father had high blood pressure, but that was when he was getting old."

"One or two relatives with these things isn't bad—heart and blood vessel diseases are so very common that two out of your four grandparents is almost average. But if you had several close relatives with early heart attacks, high blood pressure or strokes I would be more inclined to worry about your leg veins. One other question: do you smoke?"

"Yes, about a pack a day."

"Well, that's a kick in the tail for your circulation. But you're all right on the weight issue, which helps make up for it. I think you'll be safe enough on the pill if you take regular exercise and use leg-vein draining procedures when you're on your feet very long, although it would help if you would quit smoking, too."

The "regular exercise" element isn't too hard for most women of child-bearing age. Just taking care of the family's needs usually does the trick. If you're particularly sedentary, though, the habit of a daily walk (perhaps with a child or a dog) helps a lot. The "leg vein drainage" is explained in detail in Chapter Thirteen and should be used when you're standing still for any prolonged period or when you have been on your feet long enough to suffer leg discomforts. The "quit smoking" suggestion isn't really a matter of using any opening wedge to preach my little sermon: there is definite evidence that leg vein clots are substantially more common in cigarette smokers than in nonsmokers, and this difference is actually about as great as that occasioned by "the pill." A woman who quits smoking and continues the pill probably has the same or less risk from clots as one who keeps on smoking and quits the pill. One helpful technique, if you want to go this route, is spelled out in detail in Chapter Fifteen.

Cycle-confusing pills. After pregnancy pretense pills proved so successful, an entirely different type of birth control pill came into being. These "sequential varieties" are more natural in the sense that they involve almost the same amounts of almost the same hormones every fertile woman puts into her own system each month, but in a slightly different time sequence. Normally, the ovary signals the pituitary gland at the time one egg cell is released, and the pituitary signals the ovary when it is time to let another egg cell ripen. Sequential birth control pills throw off the signal system's timing so that the ovary never gets that signal and never gets an egg cell ready for fertilization.

This approach generally eliminates most side effects, including interference with sexual desire or responsiveness. Menstrual periods are usually very close to true normal (and not as light as the diminished bleeding of pregnancy pretense pills). The program is slightly more complicated to follow, however. Instead of taking one pill for twenty days, then none for the rest of the month (as witn pregnancy pretense pills), you take white pills for fifteen days, peach (or some other color) for five days, and none for eight days. Both varieties of pill are "prescription only." You will have to see your doctor to get them, and he can help you to choose the exact preparation which suits you best.

SURGERY

Doctors can sterilize either man or woman in ways which do not interfere with later marital relations. This is done by closing off the passages through which the sperm or the egg cells must move.

The main advantage of surgery is that it usually eliminates fertility once and for all. Its main disadvantage is exactly the same—it is so permanent that you usually can't find a way to undo it. This never seems like much of a problem at the time, but the one thing you can be sure of in life is that things will change. Sometimes the changes alter your family planning desires more than you would ever have expected. To cite cases:

> Joe and Marian had four children, which they felt was all they would ever want. After the last one was born, Marian had her doctor tie off her tubes. Three years later, two of the children were killed in an auto accident. Marian underwent two operations (both much more major than the original one) in attempts to get her fertility back, but never succeeded.

* * *

> Pete Marshall had his spermatic passages tied off partly because he figured three children was really all he wanted and partly because his wife was so thoroughly afraid of another pregnancy that she couldn't relax in bed. Three years later, his wife divorced him. When he remarried, his second wife wanted children badly, but he was never able to accommodate. His regret at having had the vasectomy was increased by the fact that hindsight (which is always 20/20) made him quite sure that his first wife's panic about more pregnancies was part and parcel of the deterioration in their marriage, and that he was "beating a dead horse when I gave up my fertility."

Permanence isn't always a drawback, though, and surgery might be the answer if lasting health reasons, advancing age or absolute certainty about the decision makes you totally confident. This degree of certainty is much more likely for an *individual* than for a *couple,* though, and I usually feel much safer in advising surgery for a husband who strongly feels that he has all the children he wants or a wife who has heart trouble and should not get pregnant than for these people's partners.

Here's what a woman should know about sterilizing procedures:

1. The simplest, least expensive and least uncomfortable way to sterilize a woman is to tie her tubes. *This can be done very easily in the first few days after childbirth, but otherwise requires a much more extensive procedure.* As long as the uterus is still enlarged so that its dome is well up in the abdomen, your doctor can make a buttonhole incision, and easily locate and tie off the crucial passages. When the uterus has shrunk back to its between-pregnancies size, a full scale abdominal operation is necessary to expose and alter it.

2. Your tubes can be tied in the course of most lower abdominal or pelvic operations without extra risk or discomfort. *The doctor will almost never suggest this, but will usually be glad to arrange it if you bring the matter up early in the planning phase.*

3. Extra surgery involves extra risk, and (slight though it may be) probably should be avoided. A doctor who finds some trumped-up reason to remove your uterus bypasses any sterilization committee consideration, makes sure that your insurance will pay his fee without question, and avoids any possible criticism. A patient who complains of "irregular period and discharge" in either conscious or subconscious desire for hysterectomy faces no qualms of conscience, no opposition from her husband, and no idle talk among the neighbors. But if a thousand women have hysterectomies instead of having their tubes tied, at least one of them might wind up unnecessarily dead.

For a man, the corresponding facts are as follows:

1. You can be sterilized without having any body part removed, with a procedure that takes about half an hour and can be done in a doctor's office (although many doctors prefer to work in a hospital as a convenience).

2. A few patients, especially those whose early training linked the rightness of marital relations with the function of fathering children, suffer some potency change on psychologic grounds. A few others blame the procedure for potency problems which develop months or years later, presumably from other causes. However, there is no physical reason for male sterilization to interfere with sex life or performance, and the vast majority of patients report no difficulty.

3. Except for hernia repair, this procedure does not combine well with other surgical procedures, so there is no reason to wait for a "two for the price of one" opportunity.

BIRTH CONTROL ROUNDUP

If your decisions were all between black and white, life would be very easy. The issues always seem to be shades of gray, though, with no sharp lines between them.

That's the way it is with birth control. You may not want to use any birth control measures at all, but you don't want thirteen children either. You don't want to interfere with natural physical contact, you don't want to meddle violently with your system's hormones, but you don't want to leave things too much to chance either. You might want to leave the whole decision to your doctor, but you know that he is bound to suggest a "prescription only" method if you go to him, so you really are making the choice when you walk into his door.

Perhaps this "round up" will help:

Desired end	Main Possiblities	Comments
Fewer children, not absolute control.	Rhythm alone	Reduces fertility to about half, requires ten days' abstinence a month.
	Rhythm with foam 8th through 20th day	About as safe as rhythm alone, no abstinence.
	Foam	Average failure rate about one per ten years. Slight (but usually tolerable) mess and bother.
Reversible but dependable control	Foam	No prescription required, immediate protection, no side effects. Failures very infrequent, but not as few as with "the pill."
	Pregnancy pretense pills	Require prescription, effect not established for several weeks. Side effects in some instances.
	Cycle-confusing pills	Require doctor's prescription, side effects less (but shorter observation time may leave some effects as yet undiscovered).
	IUD (coils etc.)	Failure rate about the same as foam, but no mess or clutter. Side effects, troublesome especially in non-mothers, often rule this method out.
Irreversible control	Surgery for wife	MUST BE ARRANGED BEFORE LAST CHILD IS BORN for maximum ease. Reversal unreliable and difficult.
	Surgery for husband	Excellent results in all respects except for ir-

reversibility and very infrequent potency impair-
ments (psychological in
origin but still real).

CHAPTER SEVENTEEN

Home Remedies During Pregnancy

Minnesota's raw-boned Nordic housewives seem built to bear children, but even they have discomforts and difficulties at times. A generation or two ago, they had to handle most such miseries for themselves. The automobile and the telephone have brought doctors within more ready range, but the tradition of self-reliance lingers on. Many Minnesota mothers depend on home remedies to ease the minor miseries of pregnancy, to keep down demands upon rushed rural doctors, and to handle those snow-bound emergencies.

RELIEF OF DISCOMFORTS OF EARLY PREGNANCY

Now that we're blessed with reasonable pain relief, most mothers would almost rather go through labor than endure the morning sickness, backache, fatigue and other miseries of early pregnancy Yet those discomforts can also be eased or avoided, some through home measures and others through medications your doctor will gladly prescribe on request.

CONSTANT TIREDNESS

When a woman has missed one period and wants to know whether or not she is pregnant, the first question I ask is: "Do you feel tired when you get up in the morning?"

If she is pregnant, she almost always answers "yes." An utterly dragged-out, weary feeling usually accompanies the first phase of pregnancy. It never lets up, and thus adds up to more aggravation for most women than the more intense but briefer stomach and back problems.

Need for extra protein. Rapid growth of tissue always saps your energy, whether that growth is part of a pregnancy, of body

244

self-repair (as after surgery), or of disease (as with tumor). Growing tissue takes the chemical building-blocks it needs out of your blood before other tissues meet their needs. Unless the protein foods you eat provide just the right amounts of each such compound, your muscles come up short of some strength-giving ingredients. So the first step to take in fighting the weariness of early pregnancy is to eat more protein-rich foods.

Cottage cheese, fruit-flavored yogurt and hard-boiled eggs usually prove most convenient. Work a serving of one of these in with a coffee break or snack at midmorning, midafternoon and bedtime for extra food energy without much pressure toward weight gain. You might have to cut down a little on bread or potatoes at meal time to make up for the extra calories, but very little—all three protein-rich items are usually considered good reduction foods. If you're slim enough to stand a few extra calories, a cup of hot chocolate made with milk instead of water contains double protein content and provides an excellent supplement.

Salt and fluid intake. Some women get the first inkling of pregnancy from some peculiar food craving. Dill pickles are the traditional favorite, but expectant mothers sometimes devour anything from potato chips to smoked oysters. The one thing all these foods have in common is high salt content, making these bizarre appetites a natural remedy for one source of early-pregnancy fatigue.

Every drop of fluid in your body has to have a certain amount of salt in it. During early pregnancy, both your tissues and your blood absorb extra amounts of fluid. You have to supply enough salt to go with this fluid or you suffer the same kind of fatigue usually brought on by heat exhaustion: your body's salt supply becomes depleted, your body chemistry upset, and your bodily tissues unable to function at full efficiency. Morning sickness sometimes adds to the problem two ways: by loss of salt-rich stomach juices and by decreased intake. Many women also cut down on salt deliberately, having heard that this step is wise (which is true in the last three months, but not in the earlier period).

For all these reasons, you often need extra salt during the early months of pregnancy. There are several ways to meet this need without taking pills. Soup or broth can be very heavily salted before it loses taste appeal. High-salt foods like ham and pretzels work into your menus quite easily. You can salt vegetables a bit more heavily. You might even consider drinking a salted commercial thirst-quencher like Gatorade in place of your usual beverage.

If you find that these measures relieve fatigue to some degree but can't quite keep up with your salt use, a few salt tablets might prove worthwhile. These can be purchased at any drugstore without a prescription. They have a tendency to upset an empty stomach, though, and should only be taken during or immediately after a meal.

Salt supplements, whether through natural food or through tablets, should not be continued past the fifth month of pregnancy without your doctor's specific consent, and should be discontinued earlier if swelling of the ankles or other signs of fluid accumulation develop.

Psychologic factors to consider. When a person who is *not* pregnant complains of fatigue starting right away in the morning, the problem is almost always emotional tension or upset rather than physical disease. Pregnancy scarcely makes you immune to such disturbances. The changes a new baby will make in your life mean new plans, new expectations, reshuffled human relationships— enough to make considerable turmoil in any woman's mind, no matter how thoroughly she welcomes prospective motherhood.

The best medicine for uneasiness about coming upheavals is generally concrete plans for handling the situation, with open discussion among all the parties concerned to make sure that the new arrangements will work out. So many times you will fret for weeks about some question like "Where can we put the baby's crib when we're already so crowded?" or "What in the world is going to happen when I have a baby depending on me morning, noon and night, and I can't give my husband all the attention he's gotten used to?" Just talking over these issues helps to take the sting out of them. Usually you find a solution, and even if you don't the problems seem less frightening when you reduce them to concrete issues instead of letting them float around in your head as vague worries and concerns.

While you're getting your problems into the open and resolving them, though, you may need a little temporary relief. A cup of tea or coffee often helps slightly, or a good hot cup of broth. If morning sluggishness gets to the point of real depression, your doctor can give considerable relief with prescription mood brighteners such as Elavil. At least, you should consult him about emotional miseries, as you would about physical ones. Even if the situation is temporary, why not get all the relief you can?

Morning sickness. In spite of its name, morning sickness happens morning, noon, or night. The only good thing about it is that you usually don't feel particularly nauseated—all of a sudden, you just have to empty your stomach. This, plus the fact that you usually feel fine as soon as you have finished and have no accompanying headache, diarrhea or fever, helps distinguish morning sickness from other stomach upsets (which can strike during early pregnancy as at any other time, and require prompt care).

The classic remedy for sickness first thing in the morning is two or three crackers and a bit of milk or juice before you even lift your head off the pillow, followed by a twenty-minute rest. This calls for a lot of pampering by the husband, which may explain some of the benefit—the feeling that someone else cares enough to get up early and treat you in this manner gives a real boost in morale. Frequent light feedings do seem to help, though, even after hubby has left for the office.

I usually tell patients never to let their stomachs get quite empty at this stage—a few crackers, a hard-boiled egg, a dish of cottage cheese and fruit, or a little bowl of broth midway between breakfast and lunch and again in the middle of the afternoon helps ward off most attacks. Shrink up your meals a bit to keep from getting fat on this program, of course.

Don't suffer with morning sickness very long without asking your doctor for his aid. New prescription medicines to fight nausea and vomiting, such as Compazine, work very well in most cases. These come in a variety of forms, from quick-acting pills to sustained-action capsules. The same medication can be used in the form of a rectal suppository to permit medication when the stomach is too queasy for swallowed pills to stay down. A phone call to your doctor usually lets you use these effective measures, making prolonged trial of nonprescription approaches somewhat unwise.

MIDDLE MONTH MISERIES

After the first three months or so, you get a different set of miseries from pregnancy. Let's take a look at the most common ones.

Backache. Whatever you thought of the miniskirt craze, it accomplished one worthy goal: by making women squat or stoop instead of bending over, miniskirts cut way down on backache during pregnancy. So my first piece of advice for this complaint is to pretend you're wearing the shortest skirt ever made and that the preacher is standing right behind you. Then you'll bend at the knees, instead of at the waist, do your lifting with your legs instead of your back muscles, and avoid many a muscular ache.

You're more likely to have backache during later pregnancies than on your first, probably because keeping house for the earlier children makes you do a lot more lifting. You can often cut down this lifting load in several ways. You can teach your toddlers to climb up on the bed instead of lifting them every time they need a change. You can carry wet wash and groceries in smaller batches. Maybe you can even shift some of the lifting tasks (like moving furniture when you clean) onto your husband, or skip them altogether for a while.

Some women get low back ache from pressure when the uterus is large enough to crowd the nearby organs but not quite large enough to ride up over the pelvic brim. This pain usually centers very low and in the middle of the back, and becomes worse as the day wears on. The knee-chest position exercise usually gives relief—kneel on the bed with your arms out at your sides and let your chest rest on the mattress. This lets gravity pull the uterus up out of the bony ring which constricts it. Hold the position for two minutes or so, and use it several times a day. Usually by the fifth month the uterus has enlarged enough that it stays up out of the pelvic area and this complaint disappears.

You'll read elsewhere in this book that people with backstrain or postural backache should never let a hollow form in their low back. Exaggeration of the low back curves puts pressure on pain nerves and aggravates almost any kind of back trouble. The weight shift of advancing pregnancy almost forces this postural change, and therefore aggravates any tendency to muscular or joint type back troubles. A well-designed obstetrical support can help relieve this situation, but it has to extend high enough on the chest to exert leverage against the rib cage to do any good. If your tendency to back trouble is reasonably mild, you may be able to avoid the need for a support by strengthening your abdominal muscles before pregnancy begins to stretch them. Two very mild exercises can be continued all the way through pregnancy without danger. One involves lying on your back and lifting your head off the floor for five seconds, resting for five seconds, lifting again and so on for about one minute. To do the other, simply lie on your back with your knees bent and your arms stretched to the side. Roll your hips slowly to the left until your knee touches the floor, then roll them to the right. Repeat ten times.

Kidney infection. When the uterus begins to crowd surrounding organs and vessels, the flow of body fluids sometimes detours in ways which allow germs from the intestine to reach the kidneys. Thus pain and tenderness high in the back, just below the bottom of the rib cage, calls for different treatment from ordinary back discomfort. Even in the absence of chills and fever and specific urinary complaints like frequency and burning, you have to assume that pain in this location is due to kidney infection.

Very mild, early complaints sometimes respond to simple internal flushing. Just drink ten glasses of water or non-cola pop (ginger ale, root beer, 7-up) a day to see whether extra urinary volume will wash away the germs. If complaints continue or become severe, see your doctor promptly—antibiotics work so well in this condition that it is foolish to delay their use.

Leg cramps. As pregnancy makes the uterus swell, that organ presses on the veins which carry blood back from the legs to the heart. This can cause poor circulation, pile-up of muscle-irritating waste products, and muscle cramps in the calves and in the feet.

You can usually get relief from a mild cramp by walking (or hobbling) a few steps. More severe cramps call for kneading through hot towels (p. 26) or for massage while soaking in a tub of lukewarm water.

Prevention of further attacks calls for quite different measures during pregnancy from those otherwise advised (such as quinine, which endangers the unborn baby). *Leg vein emptying exercises* sometimes help. Lie with your hips at the head end of the bed and your feet propped well up on the wall to allow blood to run downhill through your leg veins. Legs should be slightly bent, since tendons at the back of the knee press on the veins when your legs are absolutely straight. In this position, lift the balls of your feet away from the wall with your heels supporting leg weight, then lift your heels off the wall with the front of your foot supporting leg weight. Repeat five times on each occasion, and try to go through the whole routine three or four times a day.

Faintness when lying on your back. When you lie flat on your back, your uterus falls against the main blood vessels at the front of your spine. Toward the end of pregnancy, the pressure sometimes cuts off enough circulation in these vessels to partially empty the pumping chambers of your heart. Less blood coming *in* means less going *out,* and the drop in circulation makes you feel woozy or even makes you faint.

The solution to this problem is obviously to lie on your side instead of on your back. You get relief right away when the weight of the uterus shifts.

Worries about regaining your figure. One of my patients almost cried when I told her that she was pregnant.

"Of course I want the child," she said. "But I'm afraid I'll lose my husband in the process! He's commented so often on those ugly streaks women get after they have a baby, and on the way they lose their figures."

"I wouldn't worry too much about that," I said. "You'll have a few minor changes after you have your baby, of course. But you can keep them very slight by taking a few simple steps. You don't have to wind up with wide, ugly skin streaks, dangling breasts or twenty pounds of extra padding. And if you take a few simple precautions to avoid extreme changes, I'll bet your husband will be so happy with you for having his child that he'll never even notice the few minor alterations which occur."

Here are the precautions to take:

Weight watching, both to keep the baby from getting oversized and to get you back to normal size after delivery. You should gain no more than twenty pounds during a pregnancy if you want to get back to your original weight afterwards.

Vitamin C to keep your tissues fully elastic. Stretch marks on the breasts, thighs and abdomen occur when expansion is more rapid than the elasticity of the skin can tolerate. Vitamin C seems to increase normal stretchability and keep striae to a minimum. You might be able to get enough vitamin C from natural foods if you had citrus fruit or tomatoes (or their juices) with every meal. It's easier and cheaper to take pills, though. If you're taking a vitamin supplement, see how much Vitamin C (ascorbic acid) is already in it, and take extra Vitamin C if necessary to bring its total to 100 mgms a day.

Breast support day and night not only makes you more comfortable and helps you to sleep better, but also prevents most stretch marks on the breasts. If a mother plans to nurse her child, I tell her to buy her nursing bras as soon as her breasts begin to enlarge, at about the seventh month, and to wear one night and day. A few hours of nonsupport during lovemaking activity does no harm, of course.

HOME MEASURES AND OBSTETRICAL EMERGENCIES

From the very start of pregnancy, bleeding and pain signal possible serious trouble. While some of the causes remedy themselves, others require care quite urgently. So it isn't smart to "wait and see"—you have to take steps right away to settle the question.

Early bleeding. Pregnancy doesn't always stop menstruation cold. About one woman in five has some bleeding at the time of the first expected period, and some continue a scanty cycle for several months. There just isn't any way to tell this innocent bleeding from the start of a complication, though, so you're smart to always act as if you might be losing the baby. Even in the absence of cramps, this means that you should go to bed, avoid intercourse, and take no douches. If bleeding becomes heavier than normal menstrual flow or is accompanied by cramps, get in touch with your doctor. If you think the cramps might be due to constipation, use glycerin suppositories, mineral oil or milk of magnesia (two tablespoonsful nightly). Avoid enemas or strong cathartics (which might make the situation worse if the complaints come from threatened miscarriage).

Some of the important complications of early pregnancy can only be sorted out by a physician's tests. It isn't safe to continue with home measures for more than a day or so, or to continue them when you have substantial cramps and heavy bleeding. In these instances, get in touch with your physician right away.

BLEEDING EMERGENCIES

Whether early, midway, or late in pregnancy, any substantial bleeding should send you to your doctor or hospital right away. Any tearing loose of blood vessels or attachments between mother and unborn infant can lead quickly to substantial hemorrhage. Several home measures sometimes prove helpful, though.

When a woman starts to bleed, she usually lies down. Vaginal bleeding then seems to cease or slow dramatically, and this encourages her to continue with "wait and see" tactics. All too often, however, what has really happened is that bleeding has continued with no letup at all, but with pooling of blood inside the vagina. As soon as the victim sits up or stands, blood drains out in a gush.

Lying down is a good idea, especially if blood loss is making you giddy or light-headed, but don't pay any attention to temporary changes in the amount of blood at the body surface in deciding what to do next, and don't be frightened by apparently heavier bleeding while upright.

An ice bag over the lower abdomen sometimes helps to slow uterine bleeding. The bag should be wrapped in a towel rather than applied directly to the skin in order to prevent ice burns.

One of my osteopath friends showed me a trick for controlling uterine bleeding after normal delivery which also applies to most forms of uterine hemorrhage. He had the nurse leave a few pubic hairs at full length along the top of the shaved area. After delivery, he would simply pull out two or three of these hairs and bleeding would slow abruptly for several minutes. When bleeding became heavy again, pulling out a few more hairs slowed it almost instantaneously. While this technique leaves something to be desired to a conscious woman without pain relief, the discomfort involved in pulling out two or three hairs is not too much to accept if bleeding can be genuinely decreased, and the reflexes involved work just as well without a preliminary shave.

Heavy bleeding usually calls for hospital rather than house call care, so it's better to take the patient in than to call the doctor out. If she is in the back seat of the car where she can lie down, dizziness or fainting are less likely. A means of elevating the legs, even at the price of opening a window and hanging the feet outside, may help if dizziness, faintness or other signs of shock develop.

Steady pain. Steady pain at any time in pregnancy should always send you straight to your doctor. Either true or false labor always involves cramps, which come on at intervals and leave you perfectly comfortable in between.

Marion S. recognized the difference instinctively, with the aid of two prior pregnancies for experience.

"It's not bad, doctor," she said to me on the telephone. "But it's different from anything I ever had before. Just a steady, constant ache underneath my belly button, getting a little worse all the time."

"For how long?" I asked.

"Three or four hours."

"Come on in and we'll take a look."

Examination showed a small growth attached to Marion's uterus and twisted on its pedicle so that the circulation was cut off. In a few more hours, Marion would have been in serious trouble. Thanks to her alertness, we removed the tumor without even disturbing her pregnancy and she went on to deliver a healthy full-term infant.

In other cases, steady pain apparently at the onset of labor has proved to be from ruptured uterus, internal bleeding, or any of a dozen serious but readily remedied conditions. True or false labor, gas pains, and most other discomforts which you can afford to wait out for a few hours usually come in spasms with clear intervals between. Pain that hits and stays without letup for many minutes deserves immediate attention, even if it is mild enough that you don't need relief to survive.

How to know labor pains as true or false. When the snows fly in

Minnesota, a mad dash to the hospital for possible delivery can be a harrowing thing. Bad enough to have an unnecessary hospital bill, but much worse to risk life and limb sliding around an uncleared road only to find out it was "false labor"! So the women hereabouts have developed several ways of deciding *early* whether labor pains are "for real," some of which may help you with this same problem.

Especially in first pregnancies, the baby "shifts to the starting line" or "drops" before labor actually begins. The top of the uterus generally moves an inch or two away from the rib cage, making it easier to breathe and move. This coincides with movement of the baby's head down into the pelvis, where it usually causes more pressure on the bladder than before. Until this change occurs, you don't usually have to worry much about apparent labor pains—they almost always prove to be "false."

If you weigh yourself accurately every morning when you first get up, you will usually find an abrupt drop of two pounds or so about twenty-four hours before you go into labor. This change helps you to feel true from false labor, and also gives you a chance to clean the house "before mother comes." The test is not 100 per cent reliable, but even an extra house-cleaning or two is better than having to clean in hip boots because the membranes have ruptured or to pause every five minutes for a labor pain.

Practically everybody times pains—how long they last and how long between—as their main means of judging labor. The method works much better if you time *contractions you can feel with your hand* instead of pains. False labor involves contractions of much more varied intensity and length, but many of them are not severe enough to cause pain. True labor contractions may vary considerably in duration and interval, especially in the early phase, but once they have become genuinely painful almost every contraction leads to some degree of discomfort. Lie or sit still with one hand flat on the dome of the uterus, feeling through the abdominal wall with your palm instead of your fingertips (because repeatedly digging in your fingertips would make your tummy sore). You will feel that organ become hard and rise up away from your backbone an inch or two during contractions. After feeling for this change once or twice during a painful contraction, you will find that you can easily detect it before any pain begins. If pain follows every time or virtually every time your uterus contracts, best treat it as true labor. If contractions often start but taper off without reaching the pain point, you can afford to "wait and see."

THE FINAL RIDE TO THE HOSPITAL

The days of home deliveries by candlelight had one big advantage: the mother "stayed put" instead of dashing through the snow. Hospital care gives better pain relief, better avoidance and repair of tears, and better management of complications. However, both mother and child can almost always avoid any lasting damage even if the baby is born before you get to the hospital. If you realize that the "worst that can happen" will still almost certainly be a fairly satisfactory outcome for all concerned, you will find the final dash much less upsetting.

I usually advise patients to keep a recently ironed sheet available for their final ride, and to keep a warm blanket or two in the car. You can handle emergencies better if the mother rides in the back seat. If delivery becomes imminent, she has a tendency to grunt and push down as if she were having a bowel movement rather than breathe steadily in and out. At this point, she can usually delay the coming of the baby for one or two more contractions by breathing rapidly and deeply through the mouth (which makes it impossible to bear down) during each pain.

If the baby comes in spite of this maneuver, don't try to hold him back. Spread the clean sheet and either lie or squat so that the baby has a clean place to land. The baby's head almost always pushes some bowel contents out of the rectum just before delivery, so a separate cloth in which the husband can catch and dispose of this material is a big help in keeping the area clean. Unless the hospital is still very far away, you can usually let the baby be born, leave the cord uncut and the afterbirth still inside, and then drive on.

The baby usually will cry instantly when wrapped in a blanket (which feels quite rough to his unaccustomed skin), but if not he can usually be stimulated to cry by gentle rubbing. You may need to wipe away some mucus from his mouth and nose to clear the air passages. Some bleeding with delivery is normal, and you can usually reach the hospital on time to have professional attention for any possible hemorrhage if the mother holds the baby and the father drives on. Kneading the uterus gently through the abdominal wall and my osteopath friend's hair-pulling trick (described above) sometimes help to slow bleeding if necessary.

PREGNANCY AND MEDICATION

Before leaving the subject of pregnancy, let's consider its effect on your use of home remedies for other conditions. The thalidomide tragedy, which left thousands of babies deformed for life (especially in Europe), pointed up in scarlet letters the risk of using new and untried drugs during pregnancy. While drug regulations have been tightened a bit as a result, there is still a lot to be said for avoiding strong pills and chemicals as much as you can during pregnancy.

This shifts more of the burden onto home remedy procedures which do not use chemicals. You should probably use warm compresses on an aching head or stiff neck which you might treat with aspirin if you weren't pregnant, for instance. Cold baths and applications should not be used if headaches, swelling of the feet or other signs suggest blood pressure rise, but otherwise do no harm. Gentle type enemas (like Fleet's or salt and soda) are safe until the last six weeks unless bleeding or cramps suggest possible miscarriage. Massage and exercise usually can be used so long as you avoid undue pressure on the abdomen. I don't usually worry about preparations like aluminum hydroxide or kaopectate which stay inside the intestinal passages and have no way of reaching the baby, about ointments (except those which contain cortisone or sex hormones), or about such familiar preparations as vitamins and salt pills.

Fever sometimes causes extra trouble in an early pregnancy, so I recommend tepid water sponges whenever your temperature goes over 101° F. and alcohol sponges when it goes above 103° F. regardless of the reason. You should have a doctor's care for any such infection, of course, and he will probably discuss the details.

Index